Advance Praise

"Dr. Hess provides a great deal of information and wise advice based on a quarter-century of gynecologic practice during which he has focused on the issues and needs of menopausal women. Readers will find answers to their questions and solutions to their problems in this easily read presentation of the variety of approaches now available to help women."

—Philip Sarrel M.D.,
Professor Emeritus of OB/GYN and Psychiatry,
Yale University School of Medicine

"I am delighted that Dr. Hess has written this book as it gives thousands of women the opportunity to be under his care, a privilege that I have had for 25 years. He is willing to explore any safe method of therapy that can be beneficial to his patients, and has approached this book with the same eagerness to help, heal and nurture that he has in his daily practice. Recommending this book is akin to giving friends a special gift."

—Barbara Silver-Shumway,
a grateful patient

"I had many questions regarding herbal, hormone, and natural therapies, and Dr. Hess was always able to answer my questions. He has great compassion and empathy for his patients. I often wonder how he knows so much about menopause when he is a guy!"

—Jackie Easton RN,
a long-time patient.

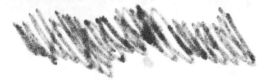

"Dr. Hess offers menopausal women a fresh approach and some new concepts I haven't seen in other menopause books [and I have read many books on this important topic]. I specifically found the suggestions on weight, wrinkles and sexuality very helpful."

—Carol Petersen RPh,CNP,
Director of Compounding and
Dispensing Operations,
Women's International Pharmacy,
Madison, Wisconsin

"Finally, women have a scientifically accurate and up-to-date resource on menopause! If you have ever been confused about the Women's Health Initiative Study, bioidentical hormones, natural approaches to menopause and many other related issues, you have bought the right book. I learned a few things myself!"

—Tara Allmen M.D.,
Columbia University College of Physicians
& Surgeons Center for Menopause
www.center-for-menopause.com

"Dr. Hess has successfully transformed 25 years of clinical practice helping his patients traverse the changes that occur with aging and menopause into an enjoyable guidebook that will now allow him to reach all women! I was especially pleased by the comprehensiveness of his chapter on sexuality. He not only normalizes the complexities of women's sexuality but provides a thorough review of potential problems and treatment options including psychotherapy, physical therapy, pharmacotherapy and herbal therapy."

—Sheryl Kingsberg Ph.D.,
Associate Professor of OB/GYN
and Chief of Behavioral Medicine,
Case Western Reserve
University School of Medicine

The Perfect
Menopause

The Perfect
Menopause

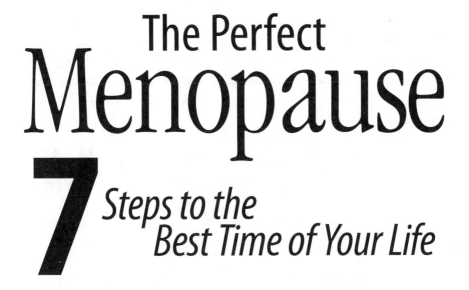

7 *Steps to the*
        Best Time of Your Life

Dr. Henry M. Hess, M.D., Ph.D.
GYNECOLOGIST, CHEMIST, NATURAL THERAPIST & MENOPAUSE EXPERT

with Tiffany Farrell

Westfall Park Publishing Group
Rochester, NY

Published by Westfall Park Publishing Group
2255 South Clinton Avenue
Rochester, New York 14618
(585) 271–7800
http://www.theperfectmenopause.com

ISBN–13: 978–1–60402–935–2 (softcover)
ISBN–13: 978–1–60402–936–9 (ebook)

Cover and Interior Design: Desktop Miracles, Inc.
Printed in the United States of America

Publisher's Cataloging-In-Publication Data
(Prepared by The Donohue Group, Inc.)

Hess, Henry M.
    The perfect menopause : 7 steps to the best time of your life / Dr. Henry M. Hess ; with Tiffany Farrell.
        p. : ill., charts ;   cm.
    Includes bibliographical references and index.
    ISBN: 978-1-60402-935-2 (pbk.)
    ISBN: 978-1-60402-936-9 (ebook)
    1. Menopause.   2. Middle-aged women—Health and hygiene. I. Farrell, Tiffany.   II. Title.   III. Title: Menopause   IV. Title: 7 steps to the best time of your life
    RG186 .H47   2008

618.1/75

To my wife Lynn Marie,
who was there to help
right from the beginning thoughts of this book,
to the finish line.

and

To Aunt Jane and Uncle Ray,
whose lifelong enthusiastic support
was always appreciated and
who always noticed that
"the midnight oil is still burning."

Disclaimer

This book is meant to educate all women on the latest options for management of their menopause. However, it should not be used as an alternative to appropriate medical care. The information given here is designed to help you make informed decisions in the context of your specific medical situation with the help of your qualified medical provider.

In the light of ongoing research and the constant flow of information, newer medical discoveries may invalidate some of the data presented here, and could even alter the considerations discussed in this book. We hope to continue to present updated versions of this book, recognizing that "the answers will continue to change"

In view of the possibility of human error and changes in medical sciences, neither the authors, nor any individual involved in the preparation of this work for publication, nor the University of Rochester, nor any individuals or other institutions mentioned in this book warrant that the information is in every respect accurate or complete. Neither the authors, nor the University of Rochester, nor any other party or institutions mentioned in this book are responsible for any errors or omissions, or for the results obtained from the use of the information in this book. We strongly advise that the information in this book be used in collaboration with your qualified medical provider.

Table of Contents

PART 3

MORE RESOURCES TO HELP YOU ACHIEVE THE PERFECT MENOPAUSE

A Special Thank You

To the late Professor H. C. Brown, 1979 Nobel Prize laureate, and my Ph.D. professor, for his inspiration to me to pursue greatness and significance.

To Dr. Philip Sarrel, professor emeritus of OB/GYN and psychiatry at Yale University, for being my mentor in menopause, role model, and friend for many years.

To Jan Payne, my personal coach for the past year and a half, who has kept me inspired and on target while writing this book, despite the time demands of my busy clinical practice.

To Tiffany Farrell, the best medical writer in the world, who enthusiastically helped me tell my story in a clear, accurate, and inspiring way.

Foreword to Healthcare Providers

If you are a healthcare provider who cares for women at midlife, you are very likely feeling the frustration of women who come in for an annual exam with multiple questions about menopause and the associated symptoms and therapeutic options. Our patients have issues and questions too numerous to answer and resolve in the 15 to 20 minute time frame for an annual exam and complete evaluation.

I have felt that same frustration in my busy gynecologic practice.

You can't blame our patients for wanting answers, and even turning (as they have), to the Internet, friends, and health food store clerks for answers. When they come into my office, they come with books by Suzanne Somers, Dr. John Lee, or Internet articles on bioidentical hormones, often written out of context. I spend my time debating the issues rather than teaching and helping. Maybe this sounds familiar to you, too.

I know that it is hard to find good evidence-based, accurate, safe, and comprehensive materials for our patients to read prior to their visit.

I am here to help you with this.

I am a trained chemist with a Ph.D., a board certified gynecologist with more than 25 years of experience, and a trained natural therapist. I have had a career-long interest in menopause, menopause therapies, and associated hormonal problems. **Let me help you help your patients.**

I have written this book to help you, and myself, help our patients with the most accurate and up-to-date information available.

Written from my over 25 years of clinical experience, this systematic book:

- Clearly defines menopause and the menopause experience.
- Gives insight into the history of menopause therapies.
- Accurately and clearly defines and discusses bioidentical hormones.
- Provides all current options for therapies, including natural and herbal therapies, medicinal therapies, and up-to-date, safe approaches to hormone therapies.
- Clearly discusses and offers solutions for those difficult issues of perimenopausal/menopausal weight gain, sexual issues, and difficulties with sleep.

You can recommend this book to your patients with the confidence that it is clearly written, up-to-date, and offers her options—safe options. You can feel confident knowing that this book is written by one of your colleagues who has the credentials and experience you can trust, and a lifelong interest in menopause.

Ask your patients to read this book first, and then consult with you about her options. This will give her safe and real answers, and allow you to help her quickly and more effectively. And she will be very grateful to you for the safe and effective options.

I am also willing to help you to help your patients more effectively. Write to me at www.theperfectmenopause.com with your questions.

—HENRY M. HESS M.D. PH.D.

Introduction

Why I Wrote This Book

*Are you confused and frustrated about
therapies for your menopause?*

*Are you uncertain about the safety of
medical and hormonal therapies?*

*Are you unsettled about your doctor's lack of knowledge of
natural therapies, or lack of enthusiasm for you to try them?*

Are you getting different opinions that confuse you?

You are not alone! I see patients every day who can't find the answers they are searching for to help them be comfortable with their menopause.

The answers may be simpler than you think.

If you are one of these women, you are experiencing dramatic changes in yourself and your body at your perimenopause and menopause time. Hot flashes, night sweats, insomnia, increasing weight, fatigue, joint pains, skin wrinkling, hair loss, and perhaps even a dramatic loss of your passion for intimacy—does this sound familiar? Are you wondering if you will ever look and feel "yourself" ever again?

To further confuse matters, you see actresses, models, and TV personalities your age looking and feeling vigorous. Some are promoting products and therapies that they swear have made all the difference in their menopause. You wonder, "Could these be right for me?"

The research you've done on the internet, the informal polls you've taken of your friends and family, and even your chiropractor all have different opinions about what you should do, and they are probably recommending a wide variety of products for you to take.

If you are like many of your peers, your doctors are only adding to your confusion. Your gynecologist suggests standard hormones, but you wonder about their safety. Your internist or family physician is concerned about hormone therapies and recommends different drug therapies like anti-depressants. You read about new and natural bioidentical hormones, and wonder how or if they are different, and why isn't your doctor recommending them?

Does any of this sound familiar?
Why has this become so confusing?

When Professor Albert Einstein, the famous physicist, was asked why he gave the same physics exam two years in a row, he responded: "The answers have changed!" His answer is true of the ever-evolving understanding of menopause, too.

Your menopause is not your mother's menopause. It is not even your sister's. So much more is known today about all aspects of the menopause than even just a few years ago, and our knowledge and understanding will continue to grow as more and more research is conducted.

You may be surprised to learn that most doctors, even OB/GYN's, weren't trained about menopause. Even in the best OB/GYN residencies, menopause gets little formal attention. It isn't that your doctor doesn't care. Unfortunately, many medical offices in general are simply too busy in today's HMO style of practice to spend adequate time staying current with the most up-to-date understanding of menopause and therapies. Sadly, it seems that too few practitioners have the time to really address your menopause issues.

Part of the reason you are overwhelmed with opinions and therapeutic options for menopause is that this prevailing confusion is the perfect setting for entrepreneurs! They get your attention because you are still looking for solutions, and the people and places you've traditionally turned to for answers aren't providing clear ones!

WHY I WROTE THIS BOOK . . .

Every day, women just like you come into my office who are overwhelmed with information, confused about their therapeutic options, and don't know who they can trust anymore to help them get through the menopause transition. Often times they've tried a few options without finding relief, or they've found relief, but then heard something on the news that scared them and don't know what to do. So many menopausal and perimenopausal women are seeking someone, anyone, who can be their open-minded partner while they try to navigate their way through these changes.

Giving help to menopausal and perimenopausal women has been my passion for over 25 years. I have the knowledge and expertise to help you! In addition to a Ph.D. in chemistry, I am a trained gynecologist, natural therapist, and nationally certified menopause practitioner. I believe in the mind-body-spirit approach. I have over 25 years experience in helping women like you manage their menopause successfully, naturally, and safely.

I wrote this book because I feel that I can be that open-minded partner you've been looking for to help you have the Perfect Menopause.

As you read this book you will:
- Learn what the safest and most effective options are from both medical and natural therapies.
- Learn the real facts about bioidentical hormones.
- Eliminate confusion and frustration about the many available products and therapies.
- Get pointers on how to choose and work with the perfect medical provider for you.
- Want to take action and make these the best years of your life!

We can do this together by going through the **7 steps to effectively and successfully make yours "The Perfect Menopause".** These 7 steps are designed to help you:

1. Completely understand your menopause.
2. Determine what your treatment goals are.
3. Manage your hot flashes, night sweats, fatigue, aches, and cognitive issues.
4. Stop the weight gain and release excess weight.
5. Manage your dryness, both inside and out.
6. Make dramatic improvements in your sexual desire.
7. Have a better night's sleep every night.

LET ME BE YOUR SECOND OPINION!

I wrote this book to help you understand your options. **Let me be your second opinion!** In every chapter of this book you'll find a wealth of information that will answer your questions and provide a framework for you to take action. Read this book, evaluate how this information relates to you, and then use it. Take control of this time of your life. Use the information in this book to assess your needs, options, and goals, and then share what you've learned with your medical provider. Select one who will help you choose an appropriate plan of action, and make yours "The Perfect Menopause".

KEEP IN TOUCH WITH US

Once you've read this book, please go to www.theperfectmenopause.com. Let me know about your personal menopause, and how I can help you further. Let me know what I can include in the next edition of this book that will help you. My team and I will also keep you up-to-date on the latest in menopause therapies.

One of my life's goals will be achieved if you benefit from reading this book and taking action as a result of it.

PART**ONE**

Important Facts
about Menopause

chapter

1

Do You Know This About Menopause?

- The average woman will spend one-third or more of her life in menopause.
- Menopause is new, but hormone therapy is not.
- Before 1900, most women did not live long enough to experience menopause.
- The ancients drank the urine of the young and virile men and women (hormones)—to capture the essence of their vigor and virility.
- Menopausal women in the 1800s ingested the extracts of ground up animal ovarian tissue.
- There has been significant progress made and new knowledge gained about menopause in just the last two years, all of which is relevant to your menopause management.
- Most women—even doctors—are confused by the changing data on hormone use.
- Bioidentical hormones were first isolated by chemists in 1928; they became available for general use in the 1960s.

- Bioidentical hormones are available both as compounded and pharmaceutical preparations.
- Hot flashes and night sweats are common symptoms, but the most common menopause complaints are fatigue and body aches.
- Hot flashes and night sweats last for 4–5 years for most menopausal women; for at least 10% of women, they will last for the rest of their lives.
- Weight gain, mood swings and decreased sexual desire are also common complaints at perimenopause and menopause, and there are effective ways to alleviate them.
- Weight gain is the number one complaint of women in my office practice; decreased sexual desire is the second.
- Beauty may be only skin deep. Did you know that decreased hormone levels dramatically reduce skin thickness, leading to skin dryness, wrinkling, and the rapid appearance of aging?
- Did the famous hormone study of 2002 (WHI—Women's Health Initiative) show that estrogen causes breast cancer after all? Recent analyses of this data, and additional new studies, show that estrogen use may actually prevent breast cancer for many younger postmenopausal women in at least the first five years of use.
- If you are on hormonal therapy and decide to go off, it may be risky to just abruptly stop.
- Natural doesn't necessarily mean safe. There are many natural therapies, including herbal therapies, which are safe and very useful for menopause symptoms. Some are not useful, and some may even be contaminated and/or harmful. This book will help you with these issues.
- ConsumerLab.com is a highly respected and reliable source to check on the purity of your herbal supplements.
- There are safe and effective herbs and natural substances that can help your hot flashes, night sweats, fatigue, sleep disturbance and sexual desire.
- Most medical schools and reputable OB/GYN residencies provide very little teaching and experience on menopause.

Do these facts surprise you? Read on to learn the real and current facts about menopause, and how they can affect your real options and successes for therapies.

A Brief History of Menopause Helps You Understand Your Options

YOU'VE JUST LEARNED A FEW FACTS about menopause and treatments that may have surprised you. The fact that it is only within the last century or so that life expectancies increased enough for menopause to become a regular experience for women indicates that the field of menopause is a relatively new area of medical research. Before the 1900s, the average life expectancy for women was 47. Women often died at younger ages than men because of infections and childbearing complications. Women who did live long enough to experience menopause received little support from the medical community. The few articles that were in the medical literature about menopause received little attention. At that time, the majority of doctors were male, and most of them held the Victorian view that the change of life "unhinged the female nervous system," changing women personally and physically. The implication was that menopausal women were moody, looked older, and became undesirable at menopause.

Thankfully, years of the medical community dismissing menopausal symptoms gave way to real interest and significant research. While the scientific community's understanding of the "whys, whats and hows" of menopause is still rather new, our knowledge about the experience and how to best treat the symptoms of menopause is constantly and rapidly growing. You have not been alone. Women have been living with (and through) menopause symptoms for years, and there have been long-standing efforts to deal with the experiences you are having. This is one of the big reasons that when it comes to menopause, as Professor Einstein put it, "The answers have changed."

Knowing a brief history of the medical community's research into menopause and therapies can be very helpful to you in understanding the healthcare practitioners' perspective towards recommending treatments. Appreciating their perspective may help you to communicate with him or her more effectively, and will benefit you when it comes time to carefully select your options for treatments.

PRIMITIVE AND EARLY BEGINNINGS

There are folklore stories about the kings and queens of ancient tribes who drank the urine of their young and vigorous subjects, believing it would help them stay, and feel, youthful and energetic in every way. While these ancient peoples may not have known that urine contained hormones, these are the earliest reports of hormonal therapies.

The first scientific articles in the literature about menopause treatments were seen during the 1700s. Medical practitioners suggested bloodletting as well as ingesting crushed animal parts, such as "crushed powdered penis of ass" (donkey), in an attempt to alleviate hot flashes and moodiness, symptoms ascribed to menopause even then. At that time, practitioners thought that these treatments worked. In the 1800s and early 1900s, scientific articles described "ovarian therapy" for hot flashes and moodiness. This therapy consisted of ingesting ground-up ovarian tissue from animals. Clearly, not much had changed for menopausal women in over a century!

THE FIRST HORMONE ERA (1900–1960)

By the early 1900s, considerable interest was building to understand the role of hormones during the menopause transition. A medical article published in 1903 linked the reduced level of hormones in menopausal women with symptoms such as hot flashes, however treatment options hadn't advanced much yet. "Ovarian therapy" with extracts of ground-up cow, sheep, or pig ovarian tissue was still the recommended remedy. Partially purified fluids that had been extracted from animal ovarian tissue even became commercially available treatments for menopausal symptoms.

By the late 1920s, women's life expectancies had increased enough that the menopause transition was becoming a common occurrence. Doctors began to recognize that menopause was a syndrome with a set of symptoms, and that it was directly related to a decline in estrogen production by the body. Then, in 1928, the German chemist, Butenandt, extracted the human ovarian hormone estrone from the urine of pregnant women. This was the first discovery of a "bioidentical" hormone, and Butenandt won the 1939 Nobel Prize for his discovery.

While many chemists were making good use of Butenandt's discovery, the process of extracting hormones from the urine of pregnant women simply was not a practical means to develop therapies for the increasingly large number of women who wanted to treat their menopausal symptoms. Demand for treatments was strong enough that chemists soon turned their attention to a more readily available source of hormones—animal urine. Pregnant animals, like pregnant women, excrete high levels of estrogens in their urine, however harvesting urine from pregnant animals did not pose the same practical concerns that harvesting urine from human subjects did.

Throughout the 1930s an increased intensity regarding the medical professional's concern to treat menopausal symptoms began to make its way into the medical literature. For the first time, the concept of "menopause management" was introduced, and articles recommending the use of hormones to achieve this were published.

In 1942, the first "modern" commercial hormone preparation for menopause therapy, Premarin®, was introduced into the market. Named for its source of estrogens, **preg**nant **mar**es' ur**in**e extraction, Premarin was a major

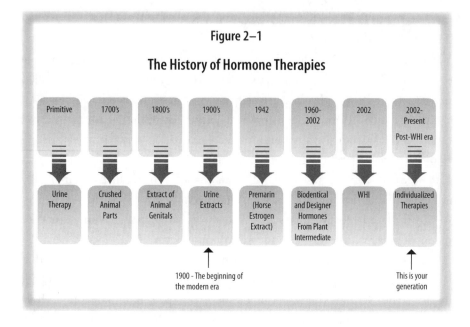

Figure 2–1

The History of Hormone Therapies

Primitive	1700's	1800's	1900's	1942	1960-2002	2002	2002-Present Post-WHI era
Urine Therapy	Crushed Animal Parts	Extract of Animal Genitals	Urine Extracts	Premarin (Horse Estrogen Extract)	Biodentical and Designer Hormones From Plant Intermediate	WHI	Individualized Therapies

1900 - The beginning of the modern era

This is your generation

breakthrough in 1942, a major advance in medicine, and a major and significant benefit to the field of menopause management. Premarin would eventually become the most widely prescribed drug in the United States. It is still available as a menopause therapy today, and its active ingredients are still extracted from the urine of the pregnant mare.

WHAT THE 1960S MEANT FOR MENOPAUSE: THE MODERN ERA OF MENOPAUSE THERAPIES

By the 1950s, more women were living much longer, and were now experiencing both menopause and many postmenopausal years. In 1960, Dr. Robert Wilson, a famous gynecologist, published the best-selling book *Feminine Forever* that promoted the concept of Estrogen Replacement Therapy—ERT. "The menopause woman is not normal," Dr. Wilson argued. "She suffers from a deficiency disease and needs treatment." This assessment summed up the prevailing thoughts of both patients and physicians regarding the menopause phenomenon. At the same time, however, a small but vocal minority was of the opinion that nothing should be done to treat menopausal symptoms. This school of thought professed that menopause was normal and that women should simply endure the symptoms. Many years later, both schools of thought were criticized for their all-or-nothing approaches. However, these opposing positions on the treatment of menopause set the tone for the ongoing debate over if, and how, menopausal symptoms are treated. This basic debate is echoed even today when any new information on menopause becomes available. You probably can name your friends and family members that are vehemently "pro" or "con" regarding the treatment of menopausal symptoms. Regardless of the intellectual debate, most women and their doctors were desperate for menopause therapies, and Premarin continued to be successfully used.

In the late 1960s, precise measurements of bone density became available and doctors discovered that significant bone loss began at menopause. Now doctors began to suggest taking estrogen as a way to protect against osteoporosis. Sales of Premarin soared.

A New Emphasis on Research

Intense research on hormones in the 1950s and 1960s allowed scientists to isolate a compound, diosgenin, which was discovered in and obtained from the yam plant. Diosgenin turned out to be a natural hormone "precursor," or building block. In the laboratory, diosgenin could be converted in to many hormones very simply, including the human-bioidentical estrogens estradiol, estrone, and estriol. Because diosgenin could be obtained from plants, this hormone precursor could be more readily available in large quantities, and with fewer practical concerns, than hormones extracted from pregnant animals. Diosgenin, it turned out, is also easily converted into other hormones in the lab such as testosterone, progesterone, DHEA, and cortisol. Large quantities of diosgenin were also found in cactus and soy plants as well. (Figure 2–2) These discoveries constituted a major advance in hormone science, and paved the way for the introduction of new, commercially-produced therapies for menopause.

The discovery of diosgenin and the ability to easily convert it into a variety of hormones led to a new, cutting-edge use for hormones: the birth

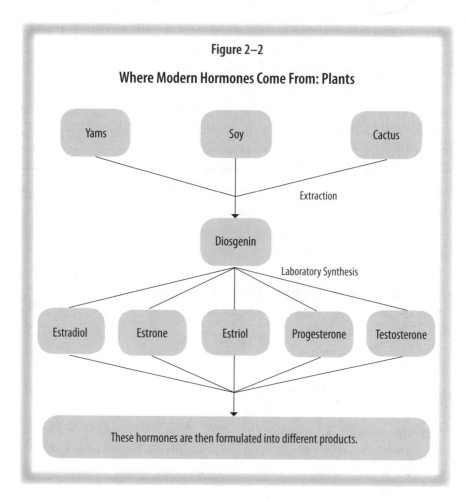

Figure 2–2

Where Modern Hormones Come From: Plants

control pill. Virtually all birth control formulations marketed today are made with a combination of synthetic estrogens and progestins produced in the lab from the hormone precursor diosgenin.

The introduction of the birth control pill in 1960 was a huge success and greatly expanded women's birth control options. A whole new sexual revolution began with the introduction of the birth control pill, and with it, a whole new era of social thinking and interactions began. Not surprisingly, the focus placed on women's health and sexuality in her reproductive years led to more interest and focus on the understanding of her menopausal years.

SOME SIDE EFFECTS OF ESTROGEN ARE EXPOSED

The latter half of the 20th century saw the most intense research and development in the area of hormones and menopause in human history. With so many women now taking hormones for their menopausal symptoms, it became easier to notice various menopause- and estrogen-related trends. Intense research showed many effects of estrogen therapies, both positive and negative. One of the most profound discoveries that has become a cornerstone of menopause therapy was that much lower doses of hormones, both in menopausal therapies and birth control pills, could be as therapeutically effective as the higher doses while decreasing the side effects. Lower-dose estrogen products quickly became the therapies of choice.

In the 1960s, menopausal women had their first "estrogen scare" when researchers reported that estrogen therapy alone (estrogen without other hormones) in women who had not had a hysterectomy may lead to an increased risk of uterine cancer. To protect the lining of the uterus, physicians added progestins to the estrogen therapy, resolving this issue for women who had not had a hysterectomy. This new treatment regimen, called combined therapy, was administered using two major treatment protocols: a combined continuous or a cyclic protocol. Combined continuous treatment, where progestin is taken every day along with the estrogen, became the most popular treatment regimen for menopausal women. In the cyclic progestin regimen, the progestin is only dosed for several days of every month or every three months. The use of progestin cyclically, instead of daily, was recommended for women who experienced unpleasant side effects from continuous progestin. Today, bioidentical porgesterone or one of the several synthetic progestins are used for this.

OTHER DISEASES AND QUALITY OF LIFE ISSUES ARE LINKED TO DECREASED ESTROGEN

Numerous women's health studies began to link estrogen deprivation at menopause to a variety of disease states. Research seemed to show that estrogen deprivation was responsible for increased risks of developing cardiovascular disease, osteoporosis, cognitive deficiencies such as memory deficits, the inability to focus, and even Alzheimer's disease. Urogenital symptoms such as bladder dysfunction, vaginal dryness and thinness, and painful intercourse were also recognized as related to the estrogen deficiency syndrome. In addition to hot flashes and night sweats, women in menopause were also widely suffering from difficulty with sleep. Sexual difficulties, including decreased libido, or sexual desire, and difficulties with orgasms, were also regarded as symptoms of estrogen deficiency at menopause.

"TAKE ESTROGEN EVEN IF YOU DON'T HAVE SYMPTOMS"

By the late 1970s through mid-2002, estrogen therapies were the hallmark of most menopause management treatment plans, and many women were put on estrogen or combination therapies either to treat significant symptoms or to prevent many of the diseases thought to be affected by estrogen loss. Even aging itself was deemed a good reason to take hormones. Many physicians in this era felt it would be malpractice not to advise patients to consider hormone therapy. Hormone therapies were extremely popular products, and the hormone preparations Premarin® and Prempro® (a combination of the estrogen-containing product Premarin and the synthetic progestin Provera®) continued to be very popular with patients and healthcare providers alike. New and alternative delivery systems containing plant-derived hormones were developed to give women more therapeutic choices and to try and further reduce the incidence of side effects. Women now can choose to take their estrogen via pills, injections, transdermal patches, skin creams and gels, or as vaginal creams, gels, rings, and suppositories. During these years, only a minority of patients requested non-hormonal alternatives to therapy, such as herbal remedies or other medicines, and few practitioners learned much about these alternatives. This minority, however, would soon be joined by thousands of women seeking a different way to alleviate their symptoms.

THE WOMEN'S HEALTH INITIATIVE (WHI) STUDY OF 2002: MENOPAUSE THERAPY UPHEAVAL

Most of you have likely read or heard reports that a major menopause-related study was stopped in 2002 because "early results showed that hormones caused cancer." How much do you know about that study? When interviewed about it, most women are unaware of the exact findings, but they often recall that it put the use of estrogen into a risky category.

The initial results published from The Women's Health Initiative Study in 2002 resulted in the first major philosophical and clinical change in the use of estrogen in many years. Suddenly, and without any warning or even a hint to the medical community, on July 11, 2002 the news media carried the story that a major, nationally-funded hormone study had been halted two years early (after only five years of study) because patients were experiencing an unacceptable increase in the risk of breast cancer. This study changed the landscape of menopause management immediately. Confusion was rampant among patients, their physicians, and even menopause experts, on how to manage menopause symptoms. Important questions about menopause and hormone therapy suddenly had conflicting answers. WHI 2002 (as I will refer to this portion of the study) forced patients and health care practitioners alike to search for wisdom on what to do about menopause and aging (I hope this book will help you in **your** search).

The WHI is indeed a large, ground-breaking study. However, the results as they were reported by the media do not tell the whole, or even the real, story of what we've learned from it. If you do not know much about the WHI study, it is extremely important that you learn about it so that you understand the status of hormone therapies today. Knowing what the WHI study was designed to discover is vitally important to your ability to properly assess the risks and benefits that discovered in the study results. Here is a brief summary:

The WHI study was designed to be a prospective, double-blind, prevention study to try to determine if two different, popular, hormone therapy regimens, as well as a vitamin-diet-lifestyle regimen, could prevent cardiovascular disease in menopausal and postmenopausal women.

A prospective study is one that tries to actively control the environment that a group of patients is subjected to in order to more directly determine a cause-effect link. Contrast this with a retrospective study, which often looks at a large number of patient charts (or in many cases, a similar endpoint that was monitored over several different prospective studies) and tries to draw conclusions about cause and effect based on what happened to patients without controlling other variables.

"Double-blind" means that the patients who were enrolled in the study either received an active drug pill, or a non-active placebo pill, and that neither the patients nor the study administrators would know which patients were on active drug and which were on placebo. Studies are "blinded" in order to remove any patient- or practitioner-held bias in favor or against the study drug. In the WHI, the active drug options were either estrogen alone for women with a hysterectomy, or continuous combined estrogen and progestin for menopausal women who still had a uterus.

A prevention study is, like it sounds, one that seeks to prevent an event. It is important to note if a study is seeking to prevent a condition as opposed to treat it. In the WHI study, researchers were attempting to prove that taking estrogen during menopause and/or in the postmenopausal years would prevent chronic diseases (primarily cardiovascular disease, secondarily cancers, osteoporosis, and dementia) as opposed to treating menopausal symptoms, such as hot flashes. This means that patients who were enrolled in the study were not necessarily required to be experiencing any menopausal symptoms at all.

Putting this all together again, the Women's Health Initiative study was designed to determine, in a bias-free environment, whether or not hormones prevent cardiovascular disease primarily, and cancer and other outcomes such as Alzheimer's, osteoporosis, and other chronic diseases secondarily, in a controlled population of menopausal and postmenopausal women. The estrogen chosen for study in women who had undergone a hysterectomy was Premarin 0.625 mg. The continuous combined estrogen-progestin study drug chosen for women who still had a uterus was Prempro, which is a combination of estrogen (Premarin 0.625 mg) and a synthetic progestin (Provera 2.5 mg).

Again, this was *not* a study designed to understand the effects of hormones or lifestyle changes in women who are experiencing menopausal symptoms (hot flashes, mood swings, etc.).

The first portion, or arm, of the WHI study to be reported on (in 2002) was the group of women who were administered either continuous combined estrogen and progestin therapy (Prempro) or placebo. This arm of the WHI study followed 16,608 menopausal or postmenopausal women aged 50 to 79 years, who did not have a hysterectomy. Half of these women were treated with placebo and half with Prempro. According to the news release in July 2002, the Prempro users, when compared to the placebo participants, developed 26% more breast cancer!

The statistics reported in the media were:

- 26% more breast cancer
- 41% more strokes
- 29% more heart attacks
- Twice as many blood clots
- 76% increase in Alzheimer's dementia
- 37% less colorectal cancer
- 33% fewer hip fractures

Over night, estrogen sounded like poison! Unfortunately, sound bites and media alerts caused great panic, and patients quit taking their estrogen therapy in droves. Given numbers like that, who wouldn't?

Most physicians, reacting to this extremely limited news, had little choice but to recommend that patients consider going off hormone therapies. Some even ordered their patients off of hormone therapies in fear of malpractice. (And malpractice lawsuits were, indeed, filed.) Ask any OB/GYN who was practicing on July 11, 2002, and they will tell you that it was a day they'll never forget. Phones were ringing off the hook. Patients everywhere didn't know what to do. OB/GYNs themselves were taken completely by surprise. And as the month progressed, the phone calls started coming in from patients who had stopped their hormones and were now begging for help to relieve their menopause symptoms. Now more than ever, patients requested alternatives, and the medical community wasn't adequately prepared.

Many previous well-designed and widely respected studies, both prospective and retrospective, which had seemingly proven the safety and benefits of hormone therapies, were suddenly discounted. Most physicians and other health care professionals, having prescribed hormone therapies safely (in their minds) for years, were not knowledgeable about alternative therapies for menopause. Remember, for years they had considered NOT prescribing hormones as near malpractice. So naturally, some health care professionals were suspicious of the efficacy and safety of alternative therapies.

STOPPING ESTROGEN SUDDENLY: THE UNACKNOWLEDGED RISK

As a result of the WHI 2002 report, either with or without the direction or urging of their physician, many women simply quit their hormone therapy. This was done despite the fact that few people (professionals or otherwise) were really aware of what the known consequences of sudden hormone withdrawal could include.

Stopping hormone therapies abruptly can cause vascular spasms. Vascular spasms occur when your blood vessels go into shock, in this case due to abrupt hormone withdrawal, which can result in sudden heart attacks or strokes. Most physicians and healthcare providers were not aware of this risk factor, and adverse outcomes did occur. The adverse outcomes from abrupt cessation of estrogen may have been far more serious than the potential negative affects that the initial data from the WHI study reported.

THE POST-WHI MENOPAUSE ERA

The WHI study is considered one of the milestones in the history of understanding menopause and menopause therapies. Once the complete data became available and was reviewed by numerous scientists, almost every aspect of the study, from its design to the interpretation of the outcomes, became intensely debated. Arguments erupted over what had really been learned in this study. Questions and criticisms were leveled at everything: the patient population, the lack of endpoints for symptom relief, author bias, the hormones and doses used, and even whether the results applied to pills alone or to alternatively-delivered hormones.

The authors of this huge, government-funded study vigorously defended the WHI. They countered that the choice of Premarin and Prempro was made because they were, by far, the most popularly used estrogen hormone therapies prescribed at the time that the study was designed (which is true). They argued that they didn't need to look at symptom relief because the goal of this study was to evaluate the role of this popular hormone therapy in the prevention of cardiovascular disease for all menopausal and postmenopausal women, symptomatic or not. And the FDA decided that the results of the WHI 2002 were applicable to all estrogen-containing menopausal therapies, regardless of formulation or delivery system. All menopausal estrogen products, whether they were alone or in combination with a progestogen, had to include what is known as a "black box" warning that outlined the results of WHI 2002.

MISLEADING RESULTS?

Many doctors and scientists felt that the way the results of WHI 2002 were presented was misleading. For example, if there were 2 cases of breast cancer in one million women and 3 cases of breast cancer in another million women, this would represent a 50% increase of breast cancer risk in the second group! The exact same data expressed in two very different ways can make a big difference in what you may believe the increased risk really is. Three versus two cases sounds much less scary than a 50% increase does, right?

26% increase in breast cancer? What did this 26%
increase in breast cancer really mean?

The actual data showed that there was an increase in the incidence of breast cancer in the group of women who were taking the continuous combined estrogen-progestin versus the women taking placebo, but only 8 more cases per 10,000 women per year. If you know that these 8 more cases are equal to a 26% increase, we can do a little math and find out that in a population of 10,000 women who take nothing for a year, approximately 31 will be diagnosed with breast cancer. That means that of 10,000 women who take Prempro® for a year, 39 will be diagnosed with breast cancer. Nobody is suggesting that any increase in cancer is good, however does 39 versus 31 cases, an increase of 8 patients in 10,000 women per year, sound as bad as a 26% increase?

Let's use a different example. Imagine that you are sitting at the beach on your beach blanket and you noticed a patch of sand on the left of the blanket where there is 10,000 grains of sand. On the right side of the blanket there is another patch with 10,000 grains. You notice there are red grains in each patch, and when you count every grain on both sides of your blanket, you find that there are eight more red grains in the right-hand patch than in the left-hand patch. If someone told you there were 26% more red grains in the second than in the first, the statistic may be correct, but a 26% increase sounds tremendously high. Without knowing what the "red-grain count" is, you might assume that there were 5000 red grains on the left, meaning there were 6300 red grains on the right (assuming a 26% increase). Or there could have been 10 red grains on the left, meaning your 26% increase equals a bit less than 3 more red grains on the right. Without a baseline number that you can calculate what "26%" is equal to in real terms, you are left to your imagination to decide if this is a slight increase or an epidemic!

WHAT DOES 8 MORE CASES OF BREAST CANCER IN 10,000 WOMEN PER YEAR REALLY MEAN?

Scientists and physicians have names for these two ways of presenting data. When using a percent, the data is being presented as a "risk ratio." When using the X cases per 10,000 patients/year, the data is called "relative risk." In clinical practice, physicians try to use relative risk as much as possible since it more accurately reflects what the real incidence of an event occurring might be in their patient population.

In 1998, the World Heath Organization (WHO) designated that the incidence of an event at 10 cases or less in 10,000 per year is a RARE EVENT, and an event of 1 case or less in 10,000 per year is an extremely rare event. Events represented as X in 10,000 per year is a standard, international way to report research findings. So an increase of 8 cases of breast cancer per 10,000 women per year that has been attributed to the use of combined therapy in menopausal women is, by the WHO definition, a rare event. The conclusion of many scientists and doctors is that the initial press coverage of the WHI 2002 study regarding breast cancer was **out of context and perspective**, leaving many women scared and with an inappropriate understanding of the issue.

THE SECOND ARM OF THE WHI STUDY—2004

The second part of the active drug portion of the WHI study was reported in 2004, nearly 2 years after the data from the first arm of the WHI was published. The second arm of the study looked at women who had a hysterectomy, and therefore took only Premarin.

The results presented of this 7-year study showed that women on Premarin alone (no progestins) had a **reduction** in breast cancer (yes, a reduction) as compared to women who had taken placebo. The relative risk was a decrease of 7 cases per 10,000 women per year, which the WHO would classify as a rare event, too. But do you remember any hype about these results? **Do these results surprise you?**

The positive results of WHI 2004 received very little attention in the media. Unfortunately, you don't get a second chance to make a first impression. Therefore, most women, and even many health care providers, remain unaware of the data that came from the estrogen-only arm of the study. They still think that estrogen causes breast cancer, and the media has devoted little attention to presenting a balanced view of estrogens based on all the information. Reductions in breast cancer, it seems, wasn't sensationally wonderful news.

The mere fact that you are reading this book means you are now aware that there is more to the WHI than what you may remember hearing about. Figure 2–3 summarizes the WHI findings, and compares the rates of relative risk found in the two arms of study. Carefully look at this figure. Your understanding of the WHI study will be much clearer, and with the appropriate knowledge of the real risks and benefits, you will be able to make informed choices about your own treatment needs.

Figure 2–3

Results of the Women's Health Initiative (WHI) Study

Outcome	2002 Prempro vs. Placebo	2004 Premarin vs. Placebo
Relative Risk Presented as: Cases Per 10,000 Women Per Year		
Breast Cancer	8 more	7 fewer
Heart Attack	7 more	No Effect
Stroke	8 more	12 more
Blood Clots	18 more	6 more
Colon Cancer	6 fewer	No Effect

*Cases per 10,000 person years is standard international method of reporting and comparing case studies.
**The World Health Organization the(WHO) has designated 10 cases or less per 10,000 patient years a RARE event.

FURTHER ANALYSES OF THE WHI STUDY

In the uproar over the WHI 2002 study report, many blanket statements and recommendations were made regarding the use of hormones that independent doctors and scientists began to question. As the media latched onto the sound bites, cooler heads were beginning to analyze and assess how specific aspects of WHI (2002 and 2004), such as patient population, choice of study drug (including formulation, dosage, and delivery system), and as we've already seen, statistical analysis, may have produced misleading recommendations about hormone use. Even in 2008, studies and analyses are ongoing to try and clarify what researchers recognized were gaping holes in our understanding of the true impact of hormones on a woman's overall health in her menopausal and postmenopausal years. In fact, about the only thing that everyone agrees upon is that hormone therapy should no longer be prescribed solely to prevent cardiovascular disease or other cardiovascular events. Nearly every other conclusion from WHI has been scrutinized to get a more specific understanding of the results likely to impact real people in a clinical situation.

Your Age Is Important

The first aspect of the WHI study to be scrutinized was the patient population, specifically the ages of the women in the study. The average woman in the study who was started on hormones was 62.5 years of age. This is 10 years older than the average age a woman usually starts a hormone therapy. In a clinical setting (the doctor's office), our typical patient who is a candidate for starting hormone therapy is the more symptomatic, early menopause woman, who is around 52 years of age. Many scientists felt that this could be an important factor affecting the outcomes of this study.

Indeed, in-depth analysis of the WHI study showed that **age does matter**. When the study was recently analyzed to specifically see the effect on women aged 50 to 59 years, there were fewer breast cancers, even in the Prempro (estrogen and progesterone) group, than in the group of women not taking hormones. Remember, the WHI 2002 arm of the study was stopped because of the increase in breast cancer! It was also discovered that, as many previous studies had shown, estrogen actually does have a protective cardio-vascular effect when started within the usual therapeutic age range—in the 50 to 59-year-old group. There seems to be a **"window of opportunity"** for prevention of cardiovascular disease when estrogen is started before age 59. Indeed, the latest 2007 version of the WHI re-analyses has shown that the risk of dying from any cause was 30% lower in hormone users in the under-59 age group. This analysis also showed that the risk of stroke and clot formation is significantly reduced when younger women, non-obese women, and women who did not have certain genetic blood clotting factors (proco-agulant or factor V Leiden) take estrogens! Transdermal estrogens were also recently found *not* to have an increased risk of blood clots, as compared to oral estrogens.

Recent Studies Shed More Light on the Estrogen/Breast Cancer Issue

In 2006, two more large, long-term studies published reports on the estrogen/breast cancer issue. The first, The Nurses' Health Study (NHS), a highly respected, long-term study that, at this printing, is still underway, reported on 28,835 postmenopausal women who have had a hysterectomy and took estrogen. The researchers stratified the outcomes by the number of years that estrogen had been used. They reported that the risk of breast cancer was not statistically significantly increased until at least 15 years of estrogen use. Additionally, in the first several years of use, a slight decrease in incidences of breast cancer was found, which is similar to the latest analyses from the estrogen-only arm of the Women's Health Initiative.

Also in 2006, a large study conducted in Finland studied the entire population of 84,729 women taking oral estrogen (in this case, mostly the bioidentical estradiol). This study also found a reduction in breast cancer in the first five years of use, similar to the results reported in WHI 2004. Slight increases in breast cancer were reported after 5 years of use, and risk increased thereafter depending on the duration of estrogen use.

A POSSIBLE REDUCTION IN BREAST CANCER IN THE EARLY YEARS OF ESTROGEN USE

These recent studies, as well as sub-analyses of the WHI itself, now show a possible reduction in breast cancer in the first five years of use and/or in the younger menopausal woman. What could be the reasons for this? The answers will likely be available in the future, but current thinking is that estrogen controls insulin levels or insulin sensitivity, a possible factor in breast cancer.

So what can you learn from all these studies? **The benefits and risks of hormone therapy depend on your individual situation.** Always keep this in mind. And don't forget Albert Einstein, "The answers have changed."

THE SUZANNE SOMERS ERA

At about the time that the WHI was making headlines in 2002, the TV actress, Suzanne Somers, hit the bookstores with her new book, *The Sexy Years*. Generally, health care providers didn't like this book, perhaps because it came at a time of confusion over the WHI. However, I found this book tremendously interesting and courageous.

The Sexy Years tells the story of a middle-aged woman who has breast cancer and has received treatment for it. It also tells the story of the same woman having a dreadful time with menopause symptoms. She researches all her options, and because of the resources available to her, she is able to consult with many experts in hormones, menopause, and cancer. Ultimately she decides that the potential risks associated with hormone therapies are a minimal risk to her, and weighed against their potentially tremendous benefits, she goes on them. She feels so much better that she writes a book about it. The difference in her life is tremendous, and she wants others to benefit from this. Using her celebrity, she is able to capture an audience and tell them her story.

After considering the options, Suzanne Somers chose bioidentical hormones—oral estradiol, testosterone, and progesterone. She chose a specific regimen and dose, and obtained her hormones from compounding pharmacies. She also recommended routine testing in order to regulate or titrate (change) her dose, and used salivary hormone testing to determine her dosage needs.

The Sexy Years tells the story of a patient who is hormonally unbalanced and who recognizes it. Once her hormones are balanced according to her biorhythms, she feels much better. Hers is a tremendous journey and one I can identify with, having treated many patients in this situation. I recommend that you read this book.

BIOIDENTICAL HORMONES HAVE A NEW BEGINNING

Remember that bioidentical hormones have been available for many years and can be taken via pills, transdermal patches, creams and gels, as well as vaginal creams, rings and suppositories. They are available from pharmaceutical companies as well as compounding pharmacies. The estrogen and progesterone molecules contained in each of these products, whether compounded or pharmaceutical, are the same and come from the same chemical companies.

The impact of the Suzanne Somers book may have taken a different course than what she intended. Patients flocked to their health care provider and wanted to be on the same regimen that Suzanne Somers was on. At the same time, there was some marketing of bioidentical hormones as a product unique to compounding pharmacies, with implications that they were safer than other hormone products! Of course, there were no studies or any credible data available to support these claims, and at a time when the WHI data was just coming out and confusion about best practices was rampant, many health care providers were very concerned about these concepts and patient requests.

SUZANNE SOMERS' SECOND BOOK

As if it weren't hard enough for you to figure out what to do with all the latest news and conflicting reports, Suzanne Somers published another book about hormones in 2006. Her second hormone book, *Ageless*, promotes **LARGE** doses of bioidentical hormones for menopausal women. Whereas her first book was an interesting and even helpful story about one woman's journey to find answers, *Ageless* presented what many health care professionals consider an irresponsible, possibly even dangerous, hormone protocol based on questionable "science."

Suzanne Somers interviewed 16 doctors for her new book on hormone therapy, but chose to recommend a controversial "treatment plan" created by a former actress, T.S. Wiley. Ms. Wiley's "hormone protocol" (she holds the patent rights and will license it for a fee to physicians or pharmacists) consists of using bioidentical estradiol and progesterone in a topical cream that is dosed to mimic the natural hormones produced by your body when you were 20 years old! Ms. Somers describes Ms. Wiley as an expert researcher, rather than the layperson she is, who has made a business out of promoting bioidentical hormones.

Seven prominent physicians, three of them interviewed for and quoted in her book, were so infuriated by *Ageless* that they wrote to her publisher, Crown, to register their objections. The three quoted in her book felt that their interviews had been distorted and were used out of context. They have objected that there is no discussion of safety issues and possible side effects of bioidentical hormones in general, not to mention of the high-dose Wiley formulation.

Ms. Somers stated in a published interview that she spent two years interviewing 16 doctors, and this was "like getting a Ph.D."

Things must have changed since I earned my Ph.D.!

Recently in interviews, T. S. Wiley described herself as a "molecular biologist and an excellent researcher," yet she holds only a bachelors degree in anthropology. Both Ms. Somers and Ms. Wiley have been on television programs promoting their books and formulations, and have rebuked the criticisms of established clinical scientists and researchers, including some interviewed in her book, as jealous, uninformed, and lacking understanding of "women's needs."

While Ms. Somers brought a much-needed message about treatment individualization to light in *The Sexy Years*, as we've seen from the re-analyses and criticisms of the WHI, not every patient is the same. The regimen Suzanne Somers uses may not be right for you. **Remember, your individual situation is unique. Work with your knowledgeable and capable provider to determine your needs and the best alternatives to addressing them to achieve *The Perfect Menopause*.**

NEW AGE PHARMACEUTICALS

As I've mentioned, physicians were desperate to help their patients in the aftermath of WHI. Many patients tried herbal therapies and found that they didn't work very well for them, but they were scared to go back on hormones. Interestingly, several new studies showed that pharmaceuticals may help with menopause symptoms, especially hot flashes, night sweats, and mood swings.

The anti-seizure medication, gabapentin, marketed as Neurontin®, has shown some promise in alleviating some menopausal symptoms. In early studies, it helped reduce hot flashes and night sweats by about 50%. However, generalized fatigue is one of the major side effects.

The antidepressant medications, or SSRI drugs, especially Effexor®, Paxil®, or even Prozac®, have also been found to help reduce hot flashes, night sweats and mood swings by about 50% in some patients. Again, there are side effects which include fatigue and sexual dysfunction (potential decreased desire as well as decreased orgasms).

These drugs do have an important role in menopause management. They are currently the most useful options for women who are experiencing moderate-to-severe symptoms and who can't take hormone therapies, such as high-risk breast cancer patients, or where other natural therapies don't work. Heath care providers who don't like hormone therapies and don't like other natural therapies may favor these pharmaceutical options.

WHERE ARE WE IN 2007?

Women who come to see me for menopause advice are more confused than ever. Each new study grabs media attention and hype, and many of the studies, or at least their sound bites, contradict each other. Very few media outlets are taking the time to interpret the new data or put it into proper perspective. What can you believe? With all the media reports, actresses, health care practitioners, and entrepreneurs championing different products, treatment regimens, and even philosophies on managing your menopause, it is no wonder so many women are left seeking answers!

After experiencing limited helpfulness from natural therapies/herbal therapies, currently these options don't seem to be as popular with women. "Bioidentical hormones" now are receiving a lot of attention and hype, leading to some misinformation and misunderstanding. Women who come to see me seeking advice have read and believe that bioidentical hormones are natural, safe, and are different from pharmaceutical hormones. Sadly, even some medical practitioners don't understand the basics of these issues and give conflicting advice and opinions.

THE FUTURE

Does this history of menopause therapy help you understand where the advice you are getting from your health care professional today may be coming from?

Will it help you in your journey to choose an appropriate course of action for you? I certainly hope your answer is, **"YES!"**

You decide your future. The history of menopause research has provided us with a lot of information, and we now know that there are lots of options for symptomatic women to try. You can benefit from this information if you can put it into perspective and use it to maximize your menopause experience. The future of all therapies, not just menopause, is individualization. Using all the available information, you can come to a decision with your health care provider on what options are best for your **individual menopause management**. You will know the real facts that are crucial to your decision process, and not be confused or misled by the media hype.

chapter

3

What Are
Bioidentical Hormones?

*Do you wonder what the recent talk about
bioidentical hormones is all about?*

*And what are the differences between
natural, synthetic, and compounded hormones?
Are they different?*

IF YOU ARE CONFUSED, you are in good company. Patients who come to my office ask these questions all the time. At the October 2006 Annual Meeting of the North American Menopause Society (www.menopause.org), the country's largest society devoted to the study of menopause, special sessions were held to review and discuss these ambiguous labels which have caused so much confusion over hormone therapy.

Why the Sudden Interest in Bioidentical Hormones?

In the initial wake of the Women's Health Initiative (WHI) study in 2002, women and health experts struggled with the sudden about-face in attitude towards hormone therapies. Women who no longer felt comfortable taking hormones looked to natural and herbal therapies to help them with their symptoms. But for many of those women, herbal therapies were not working for their significant menopause symptoms. You might be one of these women who continue to search for "natural" yet effective therapies.

Natural Estrogens

Many women in the post-WHI (2002) era assumed that "natural" hormones would be better and safer alternatives to prescription hormones. Soy supplements, which contain the isoflavones genistein, daidzein, and glycitein that exert weak estrogen-like properties in humans, enjoyed a huge surge in popularity. While these are not estrogen hormones in the strict sense, many articles in natural therapy magazines have referred to them as "natural estrogens." Unfortunately, the "natural estrogens" in soy supplements frequently don't do much to help relieve many women's menopausal symptoms.

"Bioidentical" Therapies

Are you considering, or did you start, a bioidentical hormone therapy and you still aren't sure exactly what this means?

Many health care providers attributed the "risks" of hormone therapy found in the WHI study solely to Premarin® or Prempro®, the prescription hormones used in this study. These estrogen therapies were characterized as "unnatural" or "synthetic" by consumers because they are pharmaceutical products made from a horse urine extract, and because some of the estrogens in them have slightly different chemical structures than the estrogens produced in the human body.

Premarin® and Prempro® are unique therapeutic hormones in that they are the only products on the market made from horse urine extracts. In order to differentiate the hormones used in the WHI study from other hormone products, the term "bioidentical hormones" was coined, which refers to therapeutic hormones with a chemical structure that is exactly the same as those hormones made by the human body. Many women in the post-WHI (2002) era who seek a more natural approach to hormone therapy have heard about, considered, or even started therapy with bioidentical hormones.

The new focus on bioidentical hormones should lead to a new way of thinking about hormone therapies. And it will—eventually. But like anything new in our society, the term "bioidentical hormones" will often be misused and misinterpreted—at times for profit—before the appropriate role of the actual bioidentical hormones in menopausal therapy is clearly understood. In today's health and wellness environment, it is important that you have an exact knowledge of the terms. It is extremely important to know that the terms "bioidentical," "natural," and "synthetic" have different meanings, and that many providers and entrepreneurs use these terms incorrectly either inadvertently, or to make their point or sell their product.

BIOIDENTICAL DOES NOT MEAN NATURAL

The term "bioidentical" is not clearly defined by medical dictionaries. It is a relatively new term that has only recently been coined by practitioners. I believe that to enable both practitioners and patients to make informed decisions about their therapeutic options, "bioidentical" needs to be defined, and we will provide a clear definition of it here:

Definition of NATURAL: Any product whose principle ingredient is directly sourced from an animal, plant, or mineral.

Definition of BIOIDENTICAL: Those products, in this case hormones, with a chemical structure that is identical to a product produced by the human body.

Bioidentical does not automatically mean natural! This is a very important concept to understand. The two terms are being lumped together and this is misleading.

For example, the estrogen Premarin is, in fact, "natural" because it comes directly from an animal source, but it is not "bioidentical" since the chemical structures of its components are slightly different from those of estrogens produced by humans. Advertisements are now promoting Premarin as a natural hormone. These advertisements are technically correct because the active hormones in Premarin come from an animal source. Be aware, however, that the advertisers are counting on you to assume that they mean Premarin is "natural to humans." This is just one example of how the terms applied to hormones today are being used to confuse both patients and practitioners alike.

By the definitions provided above, progesterone cream and estradiol products are "bioidentical," but not "natural," because the hormones contained in these products do not come **directly** from an animal, plant, or mineral source. **This is an important distinction!** While both of these bioidentical hormones do start from plants, there is a laboratory (synthetic) step necessary in their production to make these hormones' chemical structures identical to the hormones produced by your body. This laboratory step makes the plant-derived hormones bioidentical, but not strictly natural. They are "synthetic," but synthetic does not make them bad. In this case, synthetic makes them bioidentical! Some prefer to call bioidentical hormones semi-synthetic because the intermediate does come from natural (plant) sources.

BIOIDENTICAL, NATURAL HORMONES

Bioidentical estrogens, progesterone, testosterone, DHEA and cortisol do exist in nature as produced by the human. These hormones can be obtained from the urine of humans, as the ancients did (they drank the urine) or as the chemists did (they extracted the hormones from pregnant women's urine in the 1930s). Thus, while it is possible to have bioidentical, natural hormones, imagine trying to implement this process as a viable, large-scale solution for menopausal therapy today! This is why scientists and chemists have sought other, non-human sources of estrogens for use in therapies.

ARE BIOIDENTICAL, NON-SYNTHETIC HORMONES FROM PLANTS AVAILABLE?

No. Hormones which are bioidentical to those found in humans can be made from plants, **but not directly extracted from plants.** Estrogens produced in plants are not naturally occurring with the same chemical structure as the estrogens produced by humans. They must undergo a laboratory process in order to become bioidentical hormones. In this process, hormone precursors (hormone building blocks) are extracted from the plants and then transformed in the laboratory to make a bioidentical hormone. Soy, yams and cactus plants are the principle sources of these building blocks. Each of these plant sources contains high levels of the hormone precursor **diosgenin**. Once diosgenin has been extracted from the plant, it then undergoes a simple laboratory conversion to make a bioidentical hormone.

DOES THIS MEAN ALL COMMERCIALLY AVAILABLE BIOIDENTICAL HORMONES ARE SYNTHETIC?

Yes. Bioidentical hormones **are synthetic** in the sense that a laboratory conversion is necessary to create them. Remember, though, that due to this laboratory step, these hormones are identical in structure to the hormones naturally produced by the human body and are identical to the same hormones extracted from the urine of humans. Precursors used to make today's bioidentical hormone therapies all come from plants.

ARE BIOIDENTICAL HORMONES ONLY AVAILABLE THROUGH COMPOUNDING PHARMACIES?

No. In the wake of WHI, some books and therapists began promoting "bioidentical hormones" and "compounded hormones" as synonymous, leading consumers to assume that bioidentical hormones are only available if compounded. Several books and natural therapists have created confusion about bioidentical hormones when they imply that they must be custom mixed by a compounding pharmacy. This is simply not true! **Bioidentical hormones can be found in both pharmaceutical preparations and in compounded hormones.** Reputable compounding pharmacists will help explain this to you also.

Custom compounding is useful when a physician wants to prescribe hormones in combinations, doses, or preparations (such as lozenges or suppositories) that are not routinely available as commercial preparations. Physicians may also prescribe compounded products to order hormones not yet approved by the FDA in a pharmaceutical product for women, such as testosterone or DHEA. Some internet articles claim that bioidentical hormones are natural substances and that pharmaceutical companies cannot patent them. This is also simply not true. Don't assume that you need compounded hormones if you want to take bioidentical hormones.

Bioidentical estrogens, progesterone, testosterone, and DHEA are available commercially in a wide variety of pharmaceutical and compounded products, including pills, patches, creams, and gels, as well as vaginal creams, vaginal pills, suppositories and rings. Some of these products are available as FDA-approved pharmacological preparations, and some are available through reputable compounding pharmacies.

WHAT ARE COMPOUNDED HORMONES?

Compounded hormones can be defined as hormones mixed/prepared by a pharmacist, versus pharmaceutical hormones which are mixed/prepared by a pharmaceutical company.

DO ALL BIOIDENTICAL HORMONES COME FROM THE SAME SOURCE?

Yes. Both compounding pharmacies and pharmaceutical companies get their bioidentical hormones from the same sources: large, international chemical companies which produce them from the plant-derived hormone precursor diosgenin. (See Figure 3–1) All bioidentical hormones—compounded and pharmaceutical—come from the same chemical companies and the same plant sources.

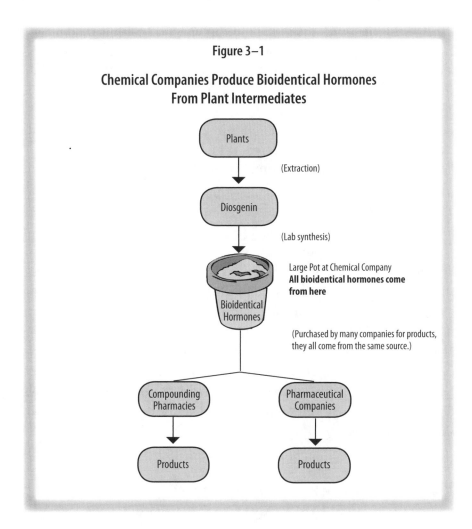

Figure 3–1

Chemical Companies Produce Bioidentical Hormones From Plant Intermediates

Plants

(Extraction)

Diosgenin

(Lab synthesis)

Large Pot at Chemical Company
All bioidentical hormones come from here

Bioidentical Hormones

(Purchased by many companies for products, they all come from the same source.)

Compounding Pharmacies

Pharmaceutical Companies

Products

Products

ARE BIOIDENTICAL HORMONES SAFER THAN OTHER HORMONES?

No one knows, but there are a large number of studies being conducted to answer this, and many other questions. Some studies are beginning to suggest that bioidentical progesterone is safer than synthetic progestins. But don't assume bioidentical hormones are safer just because of advertisements. There is absolutely no solid evidence yet that just because hormones are bioidentical they are safer than other hormone products. If you are going to take hormone therapies, it makes sense to me that you start with the bioidentical hormones. I often do that in my practice. But don't assume they are safer! Anyone who says they are safer does not have clear scientific proof and is tremendously stretching the facts.

DO COMPOUNDED HORMONES HAVE FEWER SIDE EFFECTS?

There is no evidence that compounded hormones have fewer side effects, are more effective, or are safer than pharmaceutical products containing bioidentical hormones. Be wary of anyone who makes these claims. Remember, the hormones that compounding pharmacies and pharmaceutical companies use all come from the same chemical companies and the same plant-derived hormone precursors. Compounding pharmacies have their place in menopause management. One size doesn't fit all in women's health, and compounding pharmacies help health care practitioners to individualize therapies. I use compounded hormones as well as pharmaceutical hormones for my patients. Let me say it again: **Claims that compounded hormones are safer, have fewer side effects, or are more effective just because they are compounded, simply aren't true**.

ARE COMPOUNDED HORMONES PURE, RELIABLE, AND SAFE TO USE?

In general, compounding pharmacists and pharmacies are careful, reliable and safe. There are many compounding pharmacists and pharmacies that are highly regarded and respected, and I often refer patients to these pharmacists/pharmacies. But it is important for you to know that compounding pharmacies, just by the nature of their function, are not FDA-regulated, and therefore, they are not subject to the same rules, regulations, and oversight that is applied to the pharmaceutical companies. Most states have licensing and regulatory boards for compounding pharmacies, however this type of oversight varies from state to state. Since there are no national standards, it is difficult to judge all compounding pharmacies by the same standard.

Once again, there are many excellent compounding pharmacies and pharmacists. But like all advice I am giving you in this book, do your research and choose carefully. If you are going to use a compounding pharmacy, choose one with an outstanding reputation.

ARE COMPOUNDED PREPARATIONS FDA APPROVED?

While compounding pharmacies use the same ingredients that are made into FDA-approved products, their products are currently not FDA-approved or regulated. Remember, compounded drugs are mixed to a specific order, and it is virtually impossible for there to be a national test to judge each individual preparation for dosing, consistency, or accuracy. This does not mean that that compounded drugs are unsafe. So, once again—choose a reputable compounding pharmacy.

ESTRADIOL AND ESTRIOL

While estradiol is once again regaining popularity, estriol has traditionally been the favorite estrogen hormone of compounding pharmacies and natural therapists. What exactly are these two hormones and how are compounding pharmacies using them?

The human ovary produces **estradiol,** which is the primary human estrogen. As estradiol courses through your body, it is converted into estrone (another human and bioidentical estrogen) by various body organs and tissues. Some tissues use estrone, some use estradiol, and the rate of conversion of estradiol into estrone depends on the body's needs. Estrone is a much weaker estrogen (potency) than estradiol.

Remember, though, that the menopausal woman has ovaries that are not producing much, if any, estrogen anymore. So while the predominant estrogen produced by the ovary is estradiol prior to menopause, the predominant natural estrogen in the menopausal woman is estrone.

In addition to estrone, there are several other, much weaker estrogens, that are also the products of estradiol conversion in the body. Estriol is one of these estrogens. It is a very weak estrogen (80 times weaker than estradiol) and is usually present in the body in very small amounts—except in the pregnant woman—where it is present in very large amounts.

THE TRUTH ABOUT ESTRIOL

Several years ago, some therapists assumed that since estriol is such a weak estrogen, it would be a safer estrogen to use in hormonal therapies. It was on this assumption that estriol became popular in compounding pharmacies and in compounded products. Since estriol is a bioidentical estrogen, and was available through compounding pharmacies, many practitioners found that it was a useful product to prescribe in circumstances where a very low dose or a very weak estrogen was called for. In that sense, estriol is useful, practical, and can be valuable.

As time went on, statements made in some menopause books implied that estriol even had some cancer preventative properties not found in estradiol or estrone. Unfortunately, this is clearly an extension of the facts, and there is no adequate and proven scientific evidence for these claims. Indeed, over the years there have been some case reports of uterine (endometrial) cancer and breast cancer in estriol users.

Low dose estriol vaginal cream is useful for treating thin vaginal walls (atrophy). It is available in a pharmacological cream in Europe, and as a compounded cream in the United States. Estriol may be useful when an ultra low dose estrogen is chosen. But, there is not good scientific evidence/data to show that estriol is a safer hormone or that it protects against breast cancer any differently than other estrogens.

WHAT ARE BIEST AND TRIEST?

As estriol became popular in the compounding hormone arena, specific mixtures of other bioidentical hormones also became popular. There weren't large national studies to test the safety and efficacy of this practice, but camps promoting these mixtures arose nonetheless. Biest and Triest are fairly well-defined and popularly ordered mixtures that compounding pharmacies make specifically for their clients. These mixtures were popularized a few years ago by Dr. Jonathan Wright.

The following formulas describe Biest and Triest:

Biest Mixture:	Triest Mixture:
Estriol—90%	Estriol—80%
Estradiol—10%	Estradiol—10%
	Estrone—10%

Because estradiol is so much more potent than either estrone or estriol, the major biological potency or effect of Biest and Triest in the body is probably due to the estradiol. Keep in mind that there is no scientific evidence that these products are better or safer as menopause therapies, even though they are popular mixtures available through compounded pharmacies.

WHAT ABOUT SALIVARY OR BLOOD LEVEL HORMONE TESTING TO DETERMINE WHAT HORMONES I NEED?

Some compounding pharmacies and natural therapists have promoted salivary hormone testing to evaluate and/or follow patients for hormone therapies. As a chemist, and with a 25-year history of practicing menopause/hormone management, I have carefully reviewed and studied the literature on this issue and have considerable experience with these tests. I believe that serum (blood) testing is useful in the evaluation and management of patients, but the technology simply is not there for the claim that salivary hormone levels are superior to serum (blood) hormone levels for patient management. This technology might change in the future, but for now, in my opinion, serum (blood) levels are the most accurate way to measure your hormone levels.

IS A TRANSDERMAL DELIVERY SYSTEM BETTER THAN ORAL?

Maybe. We are learning that the delivery method of estrogens is definitely important with regards to safety and efficacy. When estrogen is taken as a pill, it is absorbed in the stomach and intestines, and first processed by the liver into what the human body recognizes as "active" hormones. Once oral estrogen reaches the liver, it also stimulates the production of proteins such as C-reactive proteins, activated protein C, and clotting factors—all substances that are potentially associated with blood clots, heart disease, and stroke. This process is already different from the way the ovary produces estradiol and how that estradiol makes its first pass through the body.

Alternatively, estrogen that is delivered transdermally (through the skin) or transvaginally (through the vagina) does not need to be initially processed by the liver to be "active." Transdermal and transvaginal estrogen are both absorbed directly into the blood stream, similar to the way the ovaries release estradiol directly into the blood stream. This means transdermal delivery significantly reduces the production of the protein substances in the liver that are associated with blood clots, heart disease, and stroke. Therefore, transdermal and transvaginal estrogens may produce different effects in the body than oral estrogens.

Studies are not yet available to definitely say one route of delivery is better than the other, but studies are currently available that show a reduced risk of blood clots in women who use transdermal estrogens versus those who use oral estrogens. Studies designed to better and more thoroughly understand the possible impact that different modes of delivery can have throughout the body are currently underway. While the jury is still out, the mode of delivery—transdermal versus oral—may play an important role in determining the ultimate place of bioidentical hormones in menopausal therapy.

WHAT DO I USE IN MY PRACTICE?

For patients in my practice, I use commercially available bioidentical hormones as well as compounded hormones, depending on the situation. While not FDA-regulated, there are some excellent compounding pharmacists and pharmacies with a long history of thoroughness and exactness that I regard highly and recommend for my patients when I do prescribe compounded hormones. More specific recommendations on therapies are described in later chapters.

BE SMART ABOUT BIOIDENTICALS

I hope you have a clearer picture of what bioidentical hormones really are, and what their role in therapy might be. Having read this chapter, you should feel better equipped to discuss bioidentical hormones rationally and knowledgably with your health care practitioner, and not just follow the latest trend blindly. "Bioidentical hormones" have become such an "in thing" that in some parts of the country even chiropractors prescribe them! I have a great respect for chiropractors, but is this really their field? Hormones can be an extremely valuable component for management of your menopause, and you want an expert managing your hormone use.

As many more women enter this phase of life, there will be more and more research and more and more experts to help you manage your menopause options. But don't let entrepreneurs manage your menopause. The effectiveness and safety of your treatments depends on your knowledge about the options and forging a partnership with the right and knowledgeable provider.

PART**TWO**

The 7 Steps to the Perfect Menopause

Foreword

In the early 1500's, a young alchemist named Paracelsus worked in the mines of a well known alchemist, separating and studying the minerals extracted from ore. Alchemy is thought to be the beginning of modern day chemistry. Alchemy comes from the Egyptian words al (all) and chem (wise). As the son of a physician, Paracelsus noted the healing effects of the mineral waters on people.

Paracelsus then went on to become a physician, and using his abilities as an alchemist and physician, traveled throughout the East and Europe, often on foot. For **7 YEARS** he explored the healing effects of the substances he found in nature. Paracelsus is thought to have sowed the seeds of the beginning of homeopathy.

Like Paracelsus, I am a chemist, physician, and natural therapist. I have traveled, explored, and treated patients for over 25 years. In 1981, when I finished my residency in OB-GYN, I was already a trained chemist with a Ph.D., and had a great deal of knowledge and interest in hormones and menopause. Many patients came to see me with menopause issues and problems, and I realized that there weren't a lot of options for them. In the early 1980s, few conventional doctors really knew much about menopause. It wasn't discussed much in most residency training programs, and still isn't. This may not be a surprise to you, the menopause/perimenopause woman.

I tried to learn everything I could to help my patients with menopause problems. In addition to being a trained chemist as well as a board certified gynecologist, I studied and became an expert in natural and alternative therapies. In the last 25 years, I have traveled the world learning and teaching about all aspects of menopause therapies, and have assisted numerous patients in their search for relief of menopause symptoms and overall life wellness.

The menopause landscape has changed dramatically since I began my studies. Not only are physicians more aware of menopause issues, but many informative books on menopause are available for patients, also. Unfortunately, none of them are up-to-date with the latest options, which provide you, the patient, with a map to guide you through the options and make these years the best years of your life. Like any map, there is more than one way to reach your goal, and you need all of your possibilities presented in one place (instead of having to read multiple books and weighing their information against each other). What I've presented here is that single map with all the options drawn out for you. My patients tell me that this is what they need, and this has become my "Paracelsus" mission.

As I summarized my thoughts on how I guide patients, I realized that, over and over, my thinking came down to 7 steps. I intuitively knew that this must have some meaning or harmony, so I did a little research. The number 7 does have a special significance. There are:

- 7 days in the week
- 7 Natural Laws
- 7 creative planets in our solar system
- 7 colors in the rainbow
- 7 healing powers
- 7 chankras
- 7 spirits of God sent forth into all the earth

and many more things that come in groups of 7 that span many cultures and belief systems. It is no surprise to me that I found that my experience as a practitioner and my patients' experiences led to *The Perfect Menopause: 7 Steps to the Best Time of Your Life*.

chapter

4

Step One

Know Your Menopause

Do you wonder if you could be in menopause? What exactly are menopause and perimenopause? What should you be looking for?

DESPITE THE GREAT WEALTH of information available today, or maybe because of it, many women are confused about what menopause and perimenopause really are. Knowing what is happening to your body during these events will help you make informed choices about how you would like to approach any therapy, and make decisions about your lifestyle as you progress through these years.

THE OVARIAN CYCLE

To fully understand the nature of menopause and its impact on you, you should know the basics of the ovarian cycle. Menopause is considered the end of reproductive life; the end of childbearing function for women. The ovaries stop producing eggs (no more pregnancies) and significantly slow production of the hormones estrogen and progesterone. Menopause has been described as "ovarian failure," However this term is misleading. While the ovaries do stop egg production and most estrogen/progesterone production, they still produce a small amount of estrogen. They also continue to produce testosterone, and this function slowly declines with age, just as it does in the male testicle.

IT ALL STARTS AT PUBERTY

At birth, the human female ovary has 1 to 2 million "follicles" or tiny cysts. By puberty, the number of follicles has been reduced to between 200,000 and 400,000, and they have remained dormant until this time. At puberty (as you probably recall), lots of things change. The hypothalamic area and the pituitary gland in the brain mature and begin to send signals to the ovaries through the blood stream in the form of hormones, specifically FSH (follicle stimulating hormone) and LH (luteinizing hormone), which causes some of these follicles to mature.

MATURE FOLLICLES ARE READY FOR PREGNANCY

Stimulated by the FSH and LH signals, certain follicles in the ovaries produce an egg for potential fertilization and pregnancy. This is ovulation. During this process, these follicles also produce the hormones estrogen and progesterone (see Figure 4–1, The Ovarian Cycle). When ovarian estrogen production reaches its peak, the estrogen travels through the bloodstream back to the brain, signaling for a decrease in the flow of FSH and LH. After the lifespan of the egg-producing follicle is over (about 14 days), and if a pregnancy does not occur, the follicle begins to die. Estrogen and progesterone production also decline, marking the end of this particular "cycle," and a menstrual period begins.

The lowered level of estrogen in the blood stream signals the pituitary and hypothalamic areas of the brain to produce more FSH and LH, which

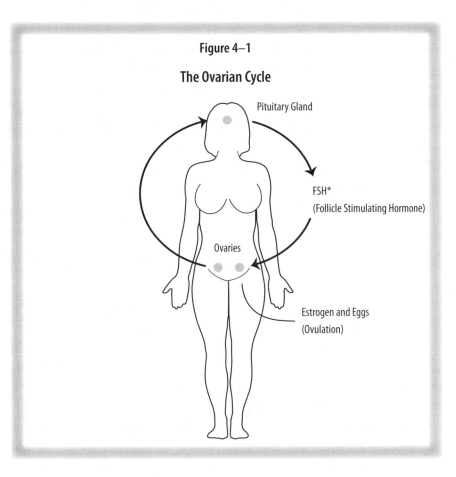

Figure 4–1

The Ovarian Cycle

Pituitary Gland

FSH*
(Follicle Stimulating Hormone)

Ovaries

Estrogen and Eggs
(Ovulation)

stimulates the ovaries anew to produce more follicles and more estrogen. Thus another cycle begins and progresses. This monthly cycle of follicle maturation, ovulation, and estrogen/progesterone production occurs from puberty until menopause. It is only interrupted by a pregnancy or an abnormality of the cyclic/ovulation process, or by taking hormones such as a birth control pill.

Low Estrogen, High FSH and LH

By the onset of menopause, most of the follicles in your ovaries have been used up or are very aged, making the ovaries unable to respond to the FSH and LH signals of the brain. There are no more ovulations, and therefore, no more estrogen and progesterone is produced. Since estrogen isn't being produced as expected, the brain increases production of FSH and LH in its continuing attempt to stimulate the ovaries. These FSH and LH signals continue to go unanswered by the ovaries, and no eggs or estrogen is produced. The concentrations of FSH and LH in your bloodstream increase to very high levels in an effort to get the ovaries to work, but the ovaries continue to be resistant to this stimulation, and thus, ovulation and estrogen production cease. Blood tests done at this time show very low estrogen levels and very high levels of FSH and LH, which is one way physicians test for menopausal status. **This is menopause!**

MENOPAUSE—ONE YEAR WITHOUT A PERIOD

Menopause is classically defined as "one year without a period." While this is the strict definition, it does not really lead to an understanding of the process. It is interesting to note that while you have been in menopause for a full year, it is only once you have completed that full year that you are officially diagnosed! Until then, the uncertainty of menopausal status can add to the frustration and confusion of this transitional time.

The average age of menopause onset is 51.4 years of age. While you may go through menopause earlier or later, most women begin between the ages of 50 and 52. Premature menopause is classically defined as beginning before age 40, and less than 1% of women experience a premature menopause. A late-onset menopause is classically defined as one that begins after age 54.5, and nearly 10 percent of women will have a late-onset menopause. Almost all women will reach menopause by 60 years old.

The hallmark of menopause is the loss of estrogen production from the ovaries and the subsequent increase in the production of FSH and LH. Short and long-term symptoms of menopause are largely related to the loss of estrogen, the increase in FSH and LH, and other factors of the natural aging process.

OTHER IMPORTANT CHANGES: PROGESTERONE AND TESTOSTERONE

In addition to estrogen, the ovaries also produce progesterone and testosterone. Progesterone is produced, along with estrogen, by the follicle during ovulation. Progesterone is produced primarily to change and nourish the lining of the uterus in preparation for a pregnancy (implantation of the fetus). When pregnancy does not occur, the progesterone levels decrease and the lining of the uterus sheds, causing a menstrual period. Because the follicles are no longer stimulated after menopause, the body stops producing most of its progesterone also. This is what contributes to the end of menstruation.

Testosterone is produced by the stromal cells in the ovaries (which do not depend on the cyclic stimulation of FSH and LH), and also by the adrenal glands. Testosterone performs many functions in your body, such as stimulating your sex drive and distributing body hair. Perhaps most importantly, it is a key driver of your overall sense of well-being. Testosterone production does not suddenly cease at menopause, as estrogen and progesterone production does. Its production decreases slowly as you age, much like it does in men. This is known as andropause, and it occurs in both men and women. Surgical removal of the ovaries, or treatment of the ovaries with drugs or x-rays, eliminates the ovarian function resulting in full cessation of estrogen and testosterone production. This causes instant menopause as well as instant andropause in women.

WHAT IS PERIMENOPAUSE?

The process of menopause can be abrupt and sudden. Your menstrual cycles may suddenly stop and symptoms of menopause begin. This isn't the usual course of events, however, unless something drastic has happened to your ovaries such as surgical removal. Usually in your 40s, you will begin to experience changes in your menstrual cycle. Your period hasn't stopped, as it does in menopause, but it becomes irregular and you may have other symptoms as well. Symptoms such as hot flashes, night sweats, mood swings, libido changes, fatigue, muscle and joint aches and pains, and vaginal dryness can occur with the menstrual irregularities, because of changes in your hormone levels. These subtle (or not so subtle) changes are called perimenopause, and they can persist for as long as 10 to 12 years before the full onset of menopause or complete cessation of your period. By definition, your peri-menopause (also referred to as the pre-menopause or menopause transition) begins at the time of variation in the menstrual cycle and ends with the last menstrual cycle.

Figure 4–2

Stages of Normal Reproductive Aging in Women

Age:	Reproductive	Perimenopause	Menopause	Postmenopausal
Periods:	Regular	Variable	No period for 1 year	Absent
FSH:	Normal	Variable	High	High
Estradiol:	Normal	Variable	Very low	Very low

CAN I STILL GET PREGNANT?

Many women will ask—if I am in menopause or perimenopause, can I still get pregnant?

The answer is a very qualified yes. It will really depend on many vari-ables. Most women don't get pregnant in their later 40s, but it still is remotely possible, and we usually recommend that patients consider using some form of birth control at least until 50. Many of my patients simply use a vaginal spermicide, as this is usually enough at this time of life. The chances of a viable pregnancy are very low at this age. For most women, pregnancy at 50 and beyond is very, very unlikely, and if it happens, most will miscarry very quickly.

Why is pregnancy still a possibility even if you haven't had a period for a year? Occasionally, for the perimenopausal woman in her late 40s or 50s, the ovary will spontaneously ovulate. This probably happens more frequently than we think. It can cause a sudden hormonal surge in a woman, and she might experience some breast tenderness, mood changes, and even a brief episode of vaginal bleeding. Or, she may not feel anything at all. When this happens, it is very normal. Very rarely, this ovulation (egg) becomes fertilized, and thus the woman would be pregnant. Mostly, however, this pregnancy would miscarry. A 50-something-year-old woman's eggs are rarely normal, and the hormonal environment in the body is rarely adequate for pregnancy implantation and nurturing.

Almost all pregnancies that you read about in women 50 and over are high-technology babies, using donor eggs and other hormonal technologies. Dr. Leon Speroff, a well-known gynecologic endocrinologist from Oregon, tells an anecdotal story of a 58-year-old woman from Oregon who naturally conceived and delivered a baby. Dr. Speroff tells the story because it can happen but it is such a rare event! In 25 years of practice, the oldest woman who naturally conceived baby I have delivered was 47 years old.

Surgical Menopause:
Hysterectomy and Oophorectomy

If your ovaries are removed in surgery (oophorectomy), menopause occurs immediately. This is where "surgical menopause" gets its name. But "surgical" menopause now has an expanded meaning due to our ability to treat some diseases without surgery. For example, if your ovaries are irradiated (x-rays) during treatment for a cancer, this may also cause the immediate cessation of estrogen production. Removal or irradiation of the ovaries also causes immediate cessation of testosterone production, too, so we could also say that women who undergo surgical menopause also experience surgical andropause. Such immediate ablation of the ovarian function leads to the instant cessation of estrogen, progesterone, and testosterone production, often with immediate and dramatic symptoms in most women.

Removal of the uterus by itself (hysterectomy) does not cause menopause unless the ovaries are removed also (sometimes called a total hysterectomy). Leaving the ovaries preserves the normal ovarian hormone function and production. However, statistics show that a woman who has had a hysterectomy (leaving the ovaries in) reaches menopause two years earlier on average. This is probably due to changes in blood flow to the ovaries as a result of the hysterectomy.

Figure 4–3

Definitions

Menopause	• Begins with the final menstrual period, but can only be recognized once a woman has gone one full year without a menstrual period. • Marks the end of reproductive life. • Marks a change in ovarian function. • Characterized by very low estrogen (estradiol) and very high FSH.
Perimenopause	• The transition years before menopause. • Characterized by period irregularity. • Other symptoms associated with the menopause may also start during this time.
Andropause	• Very low testosterone. • Usually unrelated to menopause. • Can be caused by surgical removal or other treatments to the ovaries.
Surgical Menopause	• Rapid menopause (and andropause) due to the removal of both ovaries.

Do Any Other Organs Produce These Hormones?

The adrenal glands are small glands located above each kidney and are not related to the ovaries, but they do produce sex hormones (estrogens and testosterones) in the body. During your reproductive years, the adrenal glands produce approximately half of the testosterone found in your blood stream, but they are responsible for only a very small amount of estrogen production. Hormones produced by the adrenal glands are not under the control of FSH and LH signals from the brain, and are not produced cyclically. These glands age more slowly and do not suddenly stop producing estrogen like the ovaries do.

Five Women—Different Circumstances

Where are you in your menopause? I often find that the women I see in my practice aren't sure how to answer this question. As you've seen, menopause develops and changes the longer you are in it. To help you clarify where you are in your menopause, consider these five women's stories:

Christine—53 years old—no period for seven months

Christine, 53 years old, has had very irregular periods and other menopausal symptoms since she was 46 years old. Her last menstrual period was seven months ago. She assumes she is in "menopause."

Strictly speaking, Christine is in perimenopause, or the menopause transition. Although she is beyond the age of 51.4 years, the average age of the onset of menopause, she is still within the normal age range. By classical definition, menopause begins with the last menstrual period (seven months ago) but cannot be officially declared until she has not had a period for 12 months. Her official "beginning of menopause" will then be backdated to the time of her last period. If she has another period, the clock will start over. Christine requested hormonal testing to check her menopause status. The results of her serum tests showed that her FSH was elevated and her estradiol (estrogen) was low. While this indicates that she likely has reached menopause, it is not certain until one year of amenorrhea (no period).

Karen—53 years old—no period for four years, now has bleeding

Karen, 53 years old, has not had a menstrual period since she was 49 years old. Based on one year of amenorrhea, Karen is in menopause (also referred to as postmenopause). This was confirmed by hormone testing, which showed an elevated level of FSH and a low level of estradiol.

Recently, Karen began having vaginal bleeding and wondered if this is just a "late period." **It is not!** She is clearly postmenopause. Her bleeding is abnormal and is classified as abnormal uterine bleeding, or postmenopause bleeding. Although the cause of her bleeding is likely benign, bleeding can be a sign of uterine polyps, or even cancer. A few years ago, a dilatation and curettage (commonly referred to as a D&C, or uterus scraping) would have been done. Dilatation ("D") is a widening of the cervix to allow instruments into the uterus. Curettage ("C") is the scraping of the contents of the uterus. Today, we recommend an endometrial evaluation, which examines the lining of the uterus, to determine the cause of the bleeding. Karen's endometrial evaluation includes a sonohysterogram (which is a special uterine ultrasound) and an endometrial biopsy to completely evaluate her condition.

Meg—47 years old—irregular bleeding

Meg, 47 years old, has had irregular periods for two years. She asks if she is "in menopause."

Although they are irregular, she is still having periods, which means she is in the perimenopause (or menopause transition). Hormonal testing shows her FSH and estrogen levels are variable. Although she is clearly in the perimenopause, there is no way to know how long the perimenopause will last and when she can expect her last menstrual period.

Joan—55 years old—still having periods

Joan, 55 years old, is still having menstrual periods that are more or less regular. Knowing that the average age that menopause begins is between 51 and 52, she is concerned that this is abnormal. Blood testing shows her FSH is variable, and her estradiol level is variable, too. By definition (no period for one year), Joan is not in menopause, but is in the perimenopause.

While the average age for menopause is 51.4 years, many will occur at younger ages and many will occur at older ages. There is no absolute upper age limit, although it is generally accepted that a late onset menopause is after 54.5 years of age. Approximately 10 percent of women become postmenopausal after this age. Studies are under way to see if these women with late onset menopause are at a higher risk for uterine or breast cancer. While our current knowledge does not seem to indicate an increased risk, women in this category are encouraged to have more frequent gynecologic evaluations (perhaps every six months).

Eva—47 years old—regular periods on birth control

Eva, 47 years old, was having irregular menstrual cycles and other perimeno-pausal symptoms. She was put on a low-dose birth control pill to control her very irregular bleeding and perimenopausal symptoms. She wonders how she will know when she is "in menopause."

The birth control pill, if continued, will mask the regular hormonal cycle (Refer to Figure 4–1) and will mask signs and symptoms of menopause. It will also block a true reading of her FSH and estradiol levels. In order to evaluate Eva for menopause, she will need to go off the birth control pills for a few months to see if she gets a period and to measure her FSH and estradiol levels.

Many women in this situation choose to take a very low-dose birth control pill to manage the perimenopause symptoms. These women go off the birth control pill between 50 and 53 years of age.

Do any of these women's situations sound similar to yours? Chances are good that one of them does. Remember that you are not alone. Many women before you have faced the uncertainties that come with the menopause transition, and many healthcare providers have provided guidance and assistance to them on their journeys. It is also important to remember that even though menopause is associated with a similar set of circumstances and symptoms, your combination of those circumstances and symptoms will be unique to you.

WHAT SYMPTOMS CAN I EXPECT FROM THE MENOPAUSE?

Why are the symptoms of menopause so significant? This may be because the vast majority of your organs have estrogen receptors that are affected, in some way or another, by your circulating estrogens. It is said that there are as many as 43 symptoms of menopause. The future will likely reveal many more. When estrogen levels fall, nearly all organs of the body are affected. When you are in menopause, your body is in an estrogen-deficient state. While the set of symptoms called "menopause" are primarily due to the significantly lower levels of estrogen, your decreasing levels of testosterone, perhaps progesterone and the aging process itself, are also involved.

Most women experience some symptoms of estrogen deficiency. However, your menopause symptoms and experience may be different than your friends. Menopause affects women differently. Some symptoms occur **early**, as soon as the early 40s. Other symptoms take a few years to develop, and these are referred to as **intermediate** symptoms. Some late symptoms take 10 to 20 years or more to become apparent yet are also caused by estrogen deficiency. Even though they may take many years of estrogen deprivation to become a problem, **the late symptoms of menopause are usually the most significant or most threatening to your life and lifestyle**. They will affect your overall health and longevity. Knowing what to look for with early, intermediate and late symptoms is key to developing an individualized program for the lifelong management of your menopause. Figure 4–4 provides an overview of symptoms typically associated with the early, intermediate, and late stages of menopause.

EARLY SYMPTOMS OF MENOPAUSE

You may notice early symptoms in your perimenopause time. Menstrual irregularity, irregular bleeding, or even amenorrhea (no period), are normal characteristics of the perimenopause. The most common symptoms of perimenopause and early menopause include fatigue and muscle and joint pains. Most women also experience hot flashes as well as night sweats and sleep disturbances in early menopause. About 85% of all women experience one or more of these symptoms.

Mood changes and vaginal dryness are also very common early symptoms. Increased difficulty in thinking, remembering, and mental alertness (cognitive changes) may also be experienced in the early perimenopause state. Depression, a decrease in overall well-being, or just "not feeling right," as well as a decrease in the sex drive (a decrease in libido) may also be noticed in the early menopause (or any time thereafter). Although vaginal dryness is sometimes experienced in the perimenopause and early menopause time, it occurs much more commonly after a few years of estrogen deficiency.

Figure 4–4
Symptoms of Menopause/Perimenopause

Early Menopause	• Fatigue • Joint and muscle aches • Irregular bleeding → amenorrhea (no period) • Hot flashes (flushes) • Night sweats • Mood changes, irritability • Breast tenderness • Vaginal dryness • Bloating, fluid retention • Weight gain • Memory and other cognitive changes • Sleep problems • Decrease in libido and sexual function • Decrease in overall well-being
Intermediate Menopause	• Vaginal dryness • Dyspareunia (painful intercourse) • Bladder changes and symptoms • Skin dryness
Late Menopause	• Cardiovascular disease • Cognitive issues, Alzheimer's disease • Osteoporosis • Jaw and facial bone loss • Skin aging • Eye degeneration • Tooth degeneration • General aging

---

Some women suffer greatly from these symptoms and others only experience minor discomfort or disruption. A few lucky women have no symptoms at all.

THE INTERMEDIATE SYMPTOMS OF MENOPAUSE

As menopause progresses, some symptoms that you've already been dealing with may become more significant, such as cognitive changes, sleep problems, decreased libido, and a decreased sense of overall well-being. New symptoms may also emerge as continued estrogen deprivation begins to affect other organs and body functions that rely, in some part, on estrogen.

Your vaginal and bladder walls are very sensitive to estrogen. The lowered levels of systemic estrogen associated with menopause may lead to various changes in your urogenital system, such as vaginal dryness, thinness, and decreased elasticity. In turn, these changes sometimes result in painful intercourse. Frequently, menopausal women will experience an increase of vaginal discharge and minor infections, such as yeast infections or nonspecific vaginitis, due to the dryness and thinness of the vaginal walls.

As with your vaginal walls, a deficiency of estrogen for several months or years also commonly leads to changes in bladder function. You may have more urinary urgency, frequency, or a greater need to get up in the night to go to the bathroom (nocturia). More frequent bladder infections are also a common intermediate symptom of menopause.

As time passes, the vaginal and bladder tissues thin out even more, become drier and stretch more because of estrogen deficiency. When this happens, you may develop pelvic pressure and/or some organ prolapse. Symptoms of these problems include pressure in your pelvic area, an increase in the urgency to urinate, or involuntary loss of urine with a laugh, sneeze, or during exercise.

LATE SYMPTOMS OF MENOPAUSE

While the early and intermediate symptoms of menopause are often uncomfortable and disruptive, the late menopause symptoms will have the most significant impact on your long-term health, lifestyle, and overall well-being.

Cognitive Processes: Cognitive changes during the late menopause often take the form of increased difficulty in thinking, remembering, and mentally processing information. It is likely that these changes are caused, at least in part, by a deficiency of estrogen in the brain cells themselves, as well as an estrogen-controlled decrease in the blood flow to brain cells. Recent studies show that estrogen is also involved and needed in the fluids that mediate the transmission of signals from one nerve cell to the next throughout the entire body. With the estrogen-deprived brain cells now subjected to reduced blood flow, and the ability to transmit signals from one nerve to the other hobbled, it should come as no surprise that brain functions begin to suffer. Unfortunately, the effects of reduced levels of circulating blood in the brain are linked to dementia and even Alzheimer's disease.

Cardiovascular System: In spite of recent conflicting media information, there is good scientific evidence that estrogen deficiency plays an important role in the increased risk of cardiovascular disease. Estrogen exerts a positive influence on the health and vitality of your blood vessels and it also positively affects cholesterol and lipid levels. The most recent analyses from the WHI 2002 study shows that estrogen therapy in younger menopausal women actually helped prevent cardiovascular disease. This is no small piece of news, as cardiovascular disease, not cancer, is the number one cause of death in women.

Cardiovascular disease, not cancer, is the number one cause of death in women.

Bone Density: Osteoporosis is another long-term symptom of menopause. Your bone density begins to decrease in your late 30s and early 40s, and significantly decreases at menopause. Bone loss continues throughout menopause, and has been strongly correlated with estrogen deficiency. A decrease in your bone density is thought to lead to an increased risk of osteoporosis and bone fracture.

Skin: Estrogen keeps your skin vital and healthy in a variety of ways. During menopause, your skin becomes drier, and the collagen (which makes up most of the elasticity of your skin) decreases significantly in thickness. Drying and thinning of the skin leads to wrinkling and the appearance of aging. Decreased estrogen also leads to bone loss in your facial bones. Together, these changes to your skin and bones produce an overall appearance of aging, with sunken cheeks and sagging skin.

General Aging: Inner body dryness also occurs as a result of aging, decreasing the efficiency of vital body processes. The symptoms of rheumatoid arthritis and osteoarthritis often increase, and are frequent complaints of women in perimenopause and menopause. Your teeth, gums, and eye tissue may degenerate. Blood glucose may be harder to control. All of these changes are believed to be related, at least in part, to the loss of estrogen. An increased risk for colon cancer after menopause may also be related to estrogen loss.

Research shows that many of the problems that are attributed to estrogen deficiency may be partially treatable with estrogen (See Chapters 5, 6.) Menopause experts continue to consider estrogen therapy for menopause management precisely because of its proven effectiveness at reducing or alleviating a broad range of menopausal symptoms.

MALE MENOPAUSE

Is there a male menopause? Yes, there is. Look at the end of Chapter 9 for more details.

KNOW YOUR MENOPAUSE

In Step 1, you have learned the basics of menopause. You should now understand the ovarian cycle and know what causes the estrogen deficiency associated with menopause. You are also aware that once you are in menopause, you can expect your symptoms to change over time. You have a grasp on some of the issues that many women face as they age, and will be better able to evaluate your long-term treatment goals. If you have thought through the issues presented here, then you have taken Step 1 towards achieving The Perfect Menopause.

In Step 2, we will focus on your overall profile of health and your specific menopause symptoms. You will define how your menopause is affecting you, as well as identify lifestyle choices and health considerations that will affect your options for appropriate therapy. You will also learn about the three main categories of menopause management, and probably clear up some confusion you may have about the risks and benefits of some of the options available to you.

chapter

5

Step Two

Determine Your Treatment Goals

*Are you wondering if you should take **anything** for menopause?*

*What are your symptoms, and are you
able to manage them or not?*

*Do you wonder what are the **safest**, most **effective**
methods to manage your symptoms?*

Are you like Jan?

Jan is a 52-year-old woman with significant menopause symptoms who recently consulted me. "Doctor, I'm afraid to take hormones and I'm afraid to not take them."

Or, are you like Teresa?

Teresa is a 50-year-old woman who has not had a period in two years. She has not had any menopause symptoms, but she is concerned about what she's heard about estrogen deficiency leading to chronic disease like osteoporosis. She wonders if she needs any therapy.

Or, maybe Kathy?

Kathy is 53 years old. She has not had a period in six years. During this time, she has had hot flashes so intense that her face is constantly burning, and her upper body is sweating all the time. Her night sweats are so fierce that she rarely sleeps well. The new "love handle" has been extremely frustrating, and she finds that she just isn't thinking as clearly as she used to.

Kathy's husband has been undergoing treatment for prostate cancer, so they have not been intimate in several years. Recently, her husband's physician gave him Viagra, and recommended that they resume their intimate life. "I don't know how I can," Kathy said. "My vaginal walls are so dry, I don't think it's even possible."

Kathy read Suzanne Somers' book *The Sexy Years* and saw her on *Larry King Live*. Kathy told me, "What she says makes sense to me, but then she's an actress, not a doctor. What about the articles in the *New York Times* talking about the Women's Health Initiative Study, and the dangers of estrogens? Then there are other articles, also in the *New York Times*, stating that they 'tested all the wrong women.'"

Kathy tried to research the topic on the Internet. The recommendations in the articles all conflict. "It's very confusing. One article recommends salivary testing, and another says to do something else. It puts the patient in limbo. My husband is a pharmacist, and even he is confused. I'm looking for a medical expert who is up-to-date, knows the issues, and who can help me."

LET ME HELP YOU WITH THESE DECISIONS

As we learned in Step 1, there are many symptoms associated with menopause and the menopause years. This is definitely a time in your life that demands an overall evaluation of your health. Step 2, "Determine Your Treatment Goals," provides a clear, thorough, and balanced presentation of the most up-to-date thinking on the latest treatment options for you. By the end of Step 2, you will have developed a "catalogue" of your symptoms, know which ones affect you most, and know what you might need to look out for in the future. You will have also learned about the 3 major categories (one might even say philosophies) of menopause management, and will likely have developed some thoughts about which category, or categories, you are most interested in pursuing for your own care.

HOW DO YOU BEGIN?

Begin by developing a "symptom catalogue." Start by writing down all of your symptoms. You can use the questionnaire in this book, or you can write your own list. Be thorough!

Once you've made your list, assign a "severity score" on a scale of 1 to 10 for each symptom. When I use the word severity, I am addressing two slightly different aspects of your symptoms, and I'd like you think about both of them as you are assigning a your "severity scores."

The first aspect is a rating of how bad the symptom is. Does it stop you in your tracks (a severity score of 10), or do you know you have it but you hardly notice it (a severity score of 1)? The second aspect is how manageable is the symptom? Using vaginal dryness as an example, one woman may feel like she can manage her symptoms just by using an over-the-counter lubricant (maybe a severity score of 3), while another woman has tried everything she can think of but only gets limited relief of her dryness (maybe a severity score of 8).

The scale I'd like you to use as you are assigning your severity scores are:

- 1 for "noticeable, but not bothersome" or "very manageable"
- 5 for "bothersome" or "not always manageable"
- 10 for "severe" or "unmanageable"
- Use the numbers in between, too.

Symptom	Do I have it?	Severity
Hot flashes/flushes		
Night Sweats		
Trouble falling asleep		
Trouble staying asleep		
Overwhelming urge to urinate		
Frequent urination		
Uncontrolled urination (occurring when I laugh, sneeze, etc.)		
Vaginal itching		
Vaginal dryness		
Pain with intercourse		
Dry skin		
Fatigue		
Depression		
Memory loss / mental fogginess		
Decreased libido (sex drive)		
Difficulty achieving orgasm		
Weight gain		
Joint pain		
Muscle aches		
Moodiness		
Other symptoms or situations:		

Once you have identified your symptoms and given them a severity rating, rewrite your list in order of symptom severity. Here is an example:

Symptoms	Severity
1. Fatigue	8
2. Joint and muscle aches, pains	8
3. Hot flashes, night sweats	7
4. Weight gain	6
5. Decreased libido	5
6. Disturbed sleep	5
7. Decreased memory/mental clarity	4
8. Increased moods	2
9. Vaginal dryness	1
10. Other symptoms, situations For example: (I used to love my morning coffee, but now it makes me sweat, but when I don't drink it, I feel like my work suffers because I'm not alert enough.)	7

When you show this list to your health care provider, you should know that they will see symptoms you've rated between 8-10 as clearly disabling, between 1-3 as clearly manageable. Symptoms with a rating of 4-7 will probably need to be addressed individually depending on the cause of action you take to alleviate your worst symptoms.

LIST OTHER IMPORTANT HEALTH FACTORS

Next, you need to assess other important factors such as your medical problems, and your family history of medical issues. Make sure you make note of any history of cardiovascular disease, hypertension, diabetes, hypothyroidism, elevated cholesterol, breast or other types of cancer, heart disease, and osteoporosis. Do you smoke and how much? Are you overweight? Do you exercise and how much? Do you drink alcohol or caffeine? Do you have any physical limitations? What medications are you currently taking?

The menopause and perimenopause transition is an excellent time for you to have a full physical exam and assess the entire spectrum of your health. Your family medical history and your personal health will have a significant impact on determining what menopause therapies are appropriate for you to try. It is absolutely necessary to be thorough with your health history in order to properly evaluate the benefits and risks of various therapies as they relate to you.

SET YOUR TREATMENT GOALS

Now, look at your list of symptoms and other important health factors. This is the essential information you need in order to consider what you want to achieve with therapy and optimize your outcomes. Your primary goal might be to reduce those awful hot flashes and mood swings. Or it might be to regain control over your need to get up three times a night to go to the bathroom. Either of those goals, and many others, is achievable, however the path towards achieving the one may be very different from the other! Once you know what you would like to achieve, developing a plan with your menopause expert that addresses your individual needs will be much easier.

In order to develop your plan, you must know something about the treatment options that are available to you. Gain thorough information about menopause and menopause therapies from reading this book, and use it to carefully determine your treatment goals, and to assess how you feel about the pros and cons of the different therapeutic options available to you. Write down what you see as your preferred treatment plan for you, perhaps even include multiple options in the event your first option doesn't provide the relief you hope it will.

Finally, consult with a good medical provider (refer to Chapter 11 for suggestions on how to find the right one for you) who is knowledgeable, balanced and open to all the options. Choose one who will thoroughly evaluate your total health, as well as your menopause. Your provider should help you determine a suitable management plan, and will follow up with appropriate tests and evaluations.

Treatment plans must be individualized. What works for one person may not work, or even be safe, for the next person. Don't make a quick decision when it comes to the long-term safety of your health. Your coworkers, friends, Internet connections, or health food store clerks all mean well and may be passionate about their recommendations. But they don't know all the details of your health and can not appropriately assess the safety of the products or therapies they may recommend. Be cautious and inquisitive!

Check out the story of Sue, one of my recent new patients:

Sue is a 49-year-old woman with perimenopause symptoms. She called a hotline she found on the Internet, and described her symptoms over the phone. The hotline staffer recommended she request a prescription for a "natural" hormone mixture which they assured her would be "absolutely safe." She presented this information to her internist who recommended that she consult her OB/GYN, but then wrote the requested prescription. Sue never did consult her OB/GYN. She started taking this hormone mixture, and within two months she was having heavy vaginal bleeding. A biopsy showed she had hyperplasia, which is a potential premalignant (cancerous) condition.

I don't want to scare you with Sue's story. However, I can't emphasize enough that it is extremely important to work through your treatment plan with someone who is knowledgeable about menopause, and has the credentials to back up their advice. Remember, you are going to live at least one third of your life in the postmenopause years. **Reading this book will help you end the confusion. You will know your menopause and your options.**

WHAT ARE YOUR OPTIONS?

There are three broad categories of therapies for menopause:

- Natural therapies.
- Medicinal therapies.
- Hormone therapies.

I encourage my patients to explore their feelings and beliefs about each of these categories before we make a decision about therapy. Some people want to avoid hormones or other medicines at all cost. Some people are open to all three, but wish to try the natural therapies first and move to something else if they don't work. Every woman owes it to herself to explore her feelings about the different therapeutic options. If you are uneasy with your therapeutic option, for whatever reasons, then it will be difficult to be happy with your treatment outcomes.

Explore these treatment categories thoroughly before you make decisions about what therapies are right for you. What you learn about these different categories may surprise you, and may change your mind about what is preferable or not to you. Subsequent chapters will get into greater detail about the specific regimens associated with each category addressed here. For now, I'd like to provide a broad overview of the categories for you to begin to think about.

NATURAL THERAPIES

Are you unsure about what **natural therapies** really are? Most patients who come to see me don't understand the true "nature" of natural therapies.

We learned in Chapter 3 that, strictly speaking, "natural" means "derived directly from a plant, animal, or mineral source." For example, herbs are natural therapies. We also learned that the only natural hormone product is Premarin, as it comes directly from an animal source, the urine of pregnant mares. (Never mind that it is horse estrogen.) We also learned that "bioidentical" hormones (other than those found in human urine) all come from plant precursors (themselves natural) and must undergo a synthetic process in the lab to produce a bioidentical hormone. You'll remember that "natural" does not mean "bioidentical," and that these two terms are not synonymous. If you choose to start with natural therapies, be sure you know exactly what "natural" means. **Natural does not guarantee safe!**

NATURAL THERAPIES: BEYOND HERBS

While I've defined what natural therapies are in their strictest sense, many health care practitioners use the term "natural therapy" to refer to a broader set of options that have therapeutic benefits than just those things that are "derived directly from plant, animal, or mineral sources." Most people, when referring to natural therapies, also mean lifestyle changes. Also, most people do not include Premarin in this modified definition of "natural therapies." For purposes of this book, I will use the term "natural therapies" to refer to:

- Lifestyle changes, including exercise and nutritional changes
- Herbs, vitamins, and other natural supplements
- Acupuncture, chiropractic, massage, meditation, yoga, hypnotherapy, and Tai Chi and Qigong

The range of individual responses to natural therapies varies tremendously, but I find that many patients utilizing these methods can improve their symptoms significantly. Some women who use natural therapies do not require additional therapies. Natural therapies are not only effective in treating menopause symptoms, they are often just plain healthy for you in general!

LIFESTYLE CHANGES

Menopause is the time of your life to reassess your health and to take action to improve not only your menopause symptoms, but your future health. Lifestyle changes that will improve your menopause symptoms include changes in diet and exercise. They also include quitting smoking and cutting down on alcohol and caffeine. These may seem obvious, but only reading about them won't help. You need to take action and make the change to get results. Lifestyle changes are extremely important options in menopause therapy and they are addressed individually in Chapters 6–12. **Don't bypass lifestyle changes because they seem so simple and logical.**

HERBS, VITAMINS AND NATURAL SUPPLEMENTS

Would you like to find an herb, vitamin, or other natural supplement to help relieve your menopause symptoms? Most women that I see are looking for this kind of solution, **and I think that is great! I believe in and take herbs and vitamins myself**.

Herbs are natural substances extracted from the leaves and roots of certain plants, and are generally available as capsules, teas or tinctures (an alcohol extract). Most have been used for centuries for their medicinal benefits. There are many herbs that are useful, either alone or in combination, for the reduction of many symptoms of menopause.

HAVE YOU TRIED HERBS IN THE PAST WITHOUT SUCCESS?

Many women try herbal remedies and don't achieve the relief they hoped for, but this is not a reason to give up on them quite yet! Many herbs aren't effective at first because they are taken at the wrong dose, or in the wrong combination with other herbs. Sometimes, herbal therapies don't work for the simple fact that the specific brand of herb isn't effective.

You must be cautious when you select vitamins and herbs. The FDA does not monitor most natural therapies. Some herbal products don't even have the herbal ingredients listed! And yes, the manufacturers get away with it. Herbal preparations have sometimes been found to contain contaminants, such as lead and arsenic, and their ingestion can lead to severe health problems. Cases of liver and kidney failure have been linked to contaminated herbs.

Many traditional physicians are not extensively knowledgeable about herbal products. Often, physicians are concerned about the general lack of FDA oversight and the consequences of possible contamination. This is why you get mixed messages, or even outright dismissal, from many traditional physicians about herbal products.

Take my advice as a chemist, traditional physician and natural therapist: herbs can be powerful adjuncts to menopause and other medical situations at midlife. But get expert advice on what to take. Friends, relatives, and health food store consultants don't know what is best for you, and they are not necessarily reliable resources for accurate information about herbs, herb combinations, purity, or effectiveness.

CONSUMERLAB.COM

If you and your menopause expert agree that herbs or other natural substances are an appropriate option for you, do some research on the brands that are available. I often emphasize seeking expert advice, and ConsumerLab.com is a great source of expert advice on herbal products. ConsumerLab is an independent laboratory which tests the purity and the integrity of individual brands of herbs and vitamins and publishes reports on their findings. Their findings are extremely important to you if you plan on using herbs. A subscription to this website costs approximately $30 a year. If you are serious about herbal remedies, it is money well spent to check this site before you buy a product.

HERB TO DRUG INTERACTIONS

You are aware that certain drugs can interact, even dangerously, with some other drugs. Drug-drug interactions are important considerations when you take medicines. The same is true with herbs. Some herbs can interact with other herbs and/or medicines, and cause serious effects for you. For example, many medicines and herbs can dangerously affect the action of blood thinners, either increasing or decreasing their action. If you didn't know this, this could have serious health consequences. Also, most anesthesiologists prefer that you are off all herbs for at least one week prior to having anesthesia in order to prevent any untoward interactions.

A knowledgeable provider can help you choose the correct herb or herbs, as well as brand for your particular situation. ConsumerLab.com is also an excellent resource for information on herb-herb and herb-drug interactions. Figure 5–1 is a summary of these thoughts on herbs in menopause.

Figure 5–1

Herbs In Menopause

- Truly are natural substances.
- May be helpful for menopause and other midlife health issues.
- Must be used in the correct amounts for a long enough period of time (minimum of three months) to be effective.
- Must be a reputable brand and contain the product it is supposed to contain.
- Must be pure and not contaminated.
- May need to be used in conjunction with other herbs to be effective.
- Require expert advice.
- Are milder, and therefore, tend to have fewer side effects as compared to drugs.
- Make sure the herbs won't interact with any of your other medicines.

Specific herbs are recommended throughout this book for various menopause issues. Remember, they often work, and I often consider them as first-line options for menopause therapies.

VITAMINS

Vitamins are enzymes produced by the body, or ingested in our food, that help fuel the chemical changes needed for life processes. With a good diet and a healthy body, we should have enough vitamins without taking supplements. In the 1960s and 1970s, Professor Linus Pauling, a chemist who twice won the Nobel Prize, postulated that vitamin supplements, sometimes in larger doses (for example vitamin C) may be useful for the prevention and treatment of many medical problems. Although some of Professor Pauling's postulates didn't turn out to be true, many natural and traditional medical providers believe that daily vitamin supplementation is a healthy practice. Many of our foods are not as rich as they used to be in vitamins and vitamin precursors because of poorer soils and increased utilization of processed foods, and taking vitamins helps offset this deficit.

Vitamin therapies may be useful in many menopause and perimenopause situations, either alone or in combination with herbs. But be cautious not to take vitamins in too-high doses. Some vitamins can be toxic if your dose is too high (for example, vitamin B_6). Some fat soluble vitamins (such as vitamin A) can remain in high concentrations in the body for longer periods of time. Work with your practitioner and get expert advice on how much of which vitamins to take.

OTHER NATURAL THERAPIES

Other natural therapies such as acupuncture, chiropractic, massage, yoga, Pilates, meditation, hypnosis, Tai Chi, and Qigong may be very useful and effective for relieving menopause symptoms. If they are effective for you, they may need to be practiced on a regular basis. More information will be provided regarding these therapies in Chapter 6.

MEDICINAL THERAPIES

Before 2002, women and their physicians infrequently considered non-hormonal treatments for menopause. Since 2002 (the advent of the post-WHI era), it is much more common for physicians and their patients to consider the use of medicinal or pharmacological (drug) therapies to treat significant symptoms. Medicines such as antihypertensives (example Aldomet®), antidepressants (examples Effexor®, Paxil®) and the antiepileptic gabapentin (Neurontin®) have shown the ability to reduce hot flashes, night sweats and mood fluctuations in clinical studies. Newer, shorter-acting sleeping medications such as Ambien®, Lunesta®, and Rozerem® have proven effective for sleep disturbances with minimal side effects. Medicines are also being studied to treat decreased sexual desire and weight gain.

Because these medicines are designed to have specific effects, they may be more effective than natural therapies for specific conditions. However, they may also have more potential for side effects. For example: Effexor may reduce hot flashes, night sweats and mood changes, but it also frequently causes fatigue, nausea, a decreased libido, and even weight gain in the long term. A woman considering Effexor may already be dealing with some of these known side effects as part of her set of menopause symptoms, and the last thing she may want to do is take a medicine to reduce hot flashes that could exacerbate her other menopausal symptoms! Keep in mind, though, that not everyone who takes Effexor experiences the listed side effects. Some women who can't or won't take hormones, but must take something to control those hot flashes, may experience great relief from Effexor. For them, the side effect profile might not be an issue. One size does not fit all, and with the help of your healthcare provider, you must carefully consider the pros and cons of each option when individualizing your therapy.

While medicinal therapies may be useful for certain specific menopause symptoms, and have been studied in patients who have these symptoms, none of these products carry an FDA-approved indication for the treatment of menopausal symptoms. When medicinal, non-hormonal drugs are used to treat hot flashes or night sweats, they are being prescribed "off-label." This isn't bad or wrong. Many drugs are prescribed "off-label" for a wide variety of reasons. It is important, however, that you are aware of how these medicines are being prescribed, and for what uses the FDA has studied and approved these drugs. Again, it is important to work with a menopause expert with the credentials to back up their advice when prescribing medicinal therapies for menopausal symptoms.

In subsequent chapters, medicinal therapies will be discussed for specific menopause conditions in greater detail. Medicinal therapies may be very useful for you, but consider them carefully along with all the other options. As with all therapies, they must be individualized to your specific needs and situations.

HORMONE THERAPIES

Many aspects of menopause are due to hormone-deficiency states. It is not surprising that one option to alleviate menopause symptoms, then, is to give hormones as therapies.

There is great news for you! Never has there been a time before in history where so much is known about the safety, usefulness, and risks of hormone therapies. **Estrogen in general (even in large doses) has been used safely by women for more than 75 years.** There have been many studies showing its safety and benefits. The WHI study of 2002 scared many of us, but re-analyses of the data has overturned most of the bad results. We will always be learning more about hormone therapies, **but don't overestimate the risks and underestimate the benefits**. Because of media reports, most of us tend to do this. There has never been another time when there is so much reassuring data on the use of hormone therapies.

I am sure you are wondering what the latest thinking is on hormone therapies. Are they safe, or are they poison? Are you completely opposed to hormone therapies and feel that all the issues are settled and they are unsafe? Or do you feel that hormones may have a place in the management of your menopause? And what about all the talk about bioidentical hormones?

No doubt you are frustrated by the many conflicting media reports about the effects of hormone therapies. You may be wondering how accurate, real, and relevant these reports are. There continues to be so much media attention to this issue, and so little contemplative assessment, that it is easy to be completely confused.

If you have read Chapter 2 of this book on the history of hormone therapies, you know that the WHI 2002 report made such a negative initial impact that patients went off hormone therapies in droves. In addition, many doctors, afraid of the risks of hormone therapies reported in this study, were either neutral or were urging their patients to stop taking hormone therapies.

But since the initial WHI 2002 report, there have been many re-analyses of the data from that study. These re-analyses, along with newer studies (including WHI 2004), have shown **that the answers have changed since 2002**. In the years since WHI study, a reassessment of the issue of hormone therapies has shown:

- **The culprit was Provera, not Premarin.** The WHI 2002 study used Prempro, a mixture of the estrogen Premarin and the progestin Provera (medroxyprogesterone acetate), a synthetic non-bioidentical progestin. The WHI study showed that Provera is a significant negative factor and that Provera, not Premarin, probably is responsible for many of the negative effects found in the WHI (2002). **In contrast to the negative effects of the synthetic Provera, a 2007 large study from France showed that bioidentical progesterone may reduce the incidence of breast cancer in patients taking estrogen.**

- **Premarin actually *reduced* breast cancer.** As you read in Chapter 2, WHI 2004 showed there was a reduction in breast cancer in patients who used Premarin alone without the Provera (for example, patients who had a hysterectomy). Could estrogen alone protect women from certain kinds of breast cancer? I doubt it, but researchers are wondering.

- **The study reports predominantly on the effects of estrogen in older women.** The results are different, and better, with estrogen in younger women. In the WHI study (both 2002 and 2004), patients started Prempro or Premarin for the first time at an older age. The average age of the women starting on Prempro for the first time in this study was 62.5 years of age, over 10 years past the average age of menopause onset. Recent sub-analyses of the WHI study show that when estrogen is given for the first time to the younger menopausal and perimenopausal women who participated in the WHI, there is a *protective* cardiovascular effect. This is in sharp contrast to the cardiovascular adverse effect found in the older women.

Many scientists now discuss a "window of opportunity" effect. This means that when estrogen is initiated early enough (between the mid-40s to the mid- to late-50s) there is a protective effect on the cardiovascular system, and perhaps on other systems such as the nervous system. If, however, a woman initiates estrogen long after the onset of menopause, there is a greater risk of adverse cardiovascular and perhaps other outcomes. These newer findings from the WHI suggest that estrogen has different effects, good and bad, depending on the age of the patient.

- **Transdermal estrogen behaves differently than oral estrogen.** Oral estrogen may raise triglycerides and may increase clotting factors that can lead to strokes, deep vein thrombosis, or heart attacks. Transdermal and vaginal estrogen does not raise triglycerides and does not increase clotting factors. This has a significant implication for the safety and use of estrogens.

WHAT DOES ALL OF THIS MEAN? AND WHERE DO WE STAND NOW WITH HORMONE THERAPIES?

As this book goes to press in 2008, scientists and clinicians who are experts in the field of menopause generally agree that **hormone therapy does have an appropriate place in the management of menopause and perimenopause.** Overall, it is probably the most effective therapy in the relief of hot flashes, night sweats, mood swings, and cognitive changes (lack of focus, attention, and memory). Estrogen is effective in helping treat sleep dysfunction, dryness and thinning of the skin, as well as vaginal dryness and sexual dysfunction. Hormone therapy helps to decrease fatigue, as well as muscle and joint aches and pains. It helps prevent osteoporosis, and when given early enough, helps prevent cardiovascular disease.

WHAT ARE THE SIDE EFFECTS? CAN ESTROGENS CAUSE CANCER?

This is certainly a concern of most people. Estrogens without progestins or progesterone in a woman who has not had a hysterectomy may increase the risk of uterine bleeding and even uterine cancer, so progestins or bioidentical progesterone must be used in this case. But progestins may also be the cause of the very slight increase in breast cancer incidence in some women on hormone therapies. This is one of the lessons learned from the WHI.

In order to balance these pros and cons, clinicians currently prefer to use bioidentical pgrogesterone instead of progestins, they also give the lowest effective doses of both estrogen and progesterone, and try to use progesterone as infrequently as possible (for example, protocols calling for progesterone used at intervals of only every three, or even every six, months).

Recent studies show that breast cancer risk with estrogen alone may not become significant until at least 15 years of continuous use. Risks are present for certain individuals: those who are older, heavier, and where there is a significant family history of breast cancer. Precautions such as regular breast exams and mammograms must be taken if you have one of these risk factors and choose to use estrogen.

In December 2006, there was a media story about a national reduction in breast cancer in the year 2003. The media story linked the reduction in breast cancer to the reports that women went off hormones in large numbers after the results of the WHI 2002 were published. Most patients in my practice assumed this breast cancer story was a report of a factual study. But there was no study! And there isn't any scientific data to show that the drop in breast cancer in 2003 had any relationship to estrogen use! This was pure speculation! This story failed to consider numerous other scientific facts and studies that are relevant. Consider that many women who hastily went off estrogen after WHI 2002 actually went back on hormones again because their symptoms returned. Consider also the timing: 2003 is only six months after the WHI study report, which makes a relationship between decreased usage of estrogen and a reduced breast cancer incidence unlikely. And most importantly, there are numerous potential reasons to explain the decreased national rate of breast cancer for the year 2003. It turns out that the incidence of breast cancer went down in women who never took estrogen too!

Whether or not to use hormone therapies is an individual decision and will differ for each individual. But keep in mind that hormone therapies may not be anywhere near as risky for you as you may think. **Indeed, the benefits of estrogen therapy may far outweigh the risks, especially for**

those first few years of menopause. Many of our patients choose very low-dose hormone therapies to deal with these few, very bothersome years early in menopause.

If you choose hormone therapies:

- Individualize your therapy to address your specific needs.
- Choose the lowest effective dose for the length of time appropriate to your individual needs. This may take time to discover what works best for you.
- Choose the delivery system and formulation of hormones that best fits your needs and health profile.
- Partner and work with a knowledgeable, interested, and credentialed provider.
- Monitor your therapy closely.
- Be knowledgeable and understand the latest concepts of hormone therapy. Ask questions of your healthcare provider and visit our website for updates.
- Don't jump to conclusions based on every news bulletin. Find out the facts first.

MEDIA MISINFORMATION LEADS TO UNSAFE PRACTICES

If you choose hormone therapy, be prepared for constant misinformation and incomplete information. You will be exposed to it on the news, and often from your well-meaning friends and family. Such misinformation or partial information may upset you, and disrupt your harmony. You will be tempted to stop hormone therapy based on what may not be appropriate information.

If you do want to stop taking estrogen, never stop hormone therapy abruptly. If you stop estrogen abruptly, spasms of your blood vessels are possible (which could lead to a heart attack or stroke). If you make a thoughtful decision to stop estrogen therapy, discuss this with your provider first, and develop a plan together to safely taper off.

Keep in mind that the media reports, especially with hormones, tend to be biased towards the sensational. The media know this is an emotional issue with women. Most of the time, this well-intentioned media information does not tell the whole story. Did you ever hear in the media that the second arm of the WHI study completed in 2004 showed that there was a decrease in breast cancer in the women taking Premarin without Provera?! You didn't see this splashed all over the news! It may not have been sensational to the media, but it is extremely important information for you!

DETERMINE YOUR ANSWERS

Get appropriate answers and proper guidance for your management options. Read this book carefully, make notes in the margins, and then use the information and concepts to discuss all options with a knowledgeable provider.

The next chapters, Steps 3 through 7 in the management of your menopause, will offer you options for therapies depending on your individual needs. These options, as well as thoughts and comments about them, are based on my more than 25 years of academic and clinical experience in this area. Use this information and these perspectives as a base for your thinking about your own **Perfect Menopause**.

chapter 6

Step Three
Manage Major Symptoms

ARE THE HOT FLASHES, night sweats, fatigue, aches, mood changes and brain fog a real problem for you? You are not alone! More than 85 percent of women in the perimenopause and menopause complain of one or more of these problems. Patients coming into my office often tell me these symptoms are disabling (severity scores between 8 and 10), and that they interfere with enjoying and performing daily functions. Step 3 will provide a thorough overview of the different therapeutic options you might consider in each of the three major treatment categories, and will discuss how to safely and effectively overcome your symptoms and get your life back.

HOT FLASHES AND NIGHT SWEATS

For many women, hot flashes and night sweats are the defining menopause experience. Often described as an uncomfortable wave of heat that moves through the body, leaving the face red and the body drenched in sweat, hot flashes and night sweats can be embarrassing. They can cause you to lose your concentration and disrupt your sleep patterns.

Hot flashes and night sweats typically occur multiple times within 24 hours, and usually last between one to five minutes. They can be mild, feeling only like a sensation of heat, or they can be severe and accompanied by sensations of sweating, blushing, clamminess, intense heat, and even light headedness. Symptoms are classified as mild-to-moderate symptoms if a woman has fewer than seven hot flashes in 24 hours. About one-third of women have severe symptoms, experiencing more than 10 hot flashes a day. They often begin during the perimenopause, and most women have them on and off for a few years. For many, hot flashes will dwindle and become minimal within 5 years. Perhaps as many as 10% of postmenopausal women will have hot flashes and night sweats for life.

We don't know the exact cause of hot flashes and night sweats, but we know they are related to the menopause and perimenopause. We also know that deficiencies in estrogen play a role because estrogen supplementation helps relieve the symptoms. Some scientists believe that menopause-related deficiencies in estrogen confuse the area of the brain that regulates body temperature, which is the hypothalamus. The theory is that your decreasing estrogen levels signal the thermal area of the hypothalamus to "turn up the heat." Once the "heat is on," other areas of the brain signal the body to get rid of the heat. In an effort to cool you off, blood vessels dilate in the surface of the skin, and sweat glands activate. During this process the adrenal gland activates and the resulting adrenaline rush causes palpitations (an increase in your heart rate). Some women even experience headaches and chest pain as a result of this process. Finally, the body's attempt to cool down leaves you with chills.

The estrogen-hypothalamus-hot flash connection helps us understand why estrogen works to reduce hot flashes. It also helps us understand why other medicines, such as antidepressants, and even simple methods for staying cool, work well too.

MOOD SWINGS, COGNITIVE CHANGES, FATIGUE AND ACHES

Similar brain and central nervous system mechanisms have also been suggested as the cause of increases in mood swings, as well as other transient changes such as memory deficiencies and a reduced ability to concentrate. Patients often refer to these symptoms as "brain fog."

The causes of fatigue and muscle/joint aches are less certain, but their association with menopause and hormone deficiencies is well known. Inflammation associated with chronic diseases has a relationship to lower hormone levels, especially estrogen.

Consider Christine's Story:

Christine is a 52-year-old professor at the medical school. When she was 48, she began to have hot flashes, night sweats, and noticed changes in her ability to focus and in her memory. She found herself sweating profusely during her lectures at the medical school. Even worse, she would lose her focus and concentration right in the middle of her lecture, even without a hot flash distracting her. "I couldn't continue to practice my profession," she said. "It was disabling to me."

At first, she tried vitamins and herbs, and made many significant lifestyle changes, all of which helped a great deal with the hot flashes and night sweats. She was also sleeping better, too. "But," she told me, these changes "didn't help my concentration." Christine recognized that her therapeutic goals called for something more than what natural therapies were providing, and she began to explore medicinal and hormonal therapies. After we had several discussions about the wealth of options, she told me "A lot has changed in the understanding of hormones."

Based on her research, a thorough review of her health status and family history, and our conversations, Christine opted to try a low dose of transdermal bioidentical estradiol patches. Three months later, Christine shared with me that she feels "normal again." Her cognitive issues have resolved and she feels like her "old self." Christine feels that she was "betrayed" by what she had read and heard in the last few years about hormones. She feels that the initial interpretations of the WHI study delayed the successful management of her menopause.

There are some very important lessons to learn from Christine's story. The first is that she was able to manage the majority of her symptoms with a combination of natural therapies and lifestyle changes. In this way, Christine is representative of the majority of my patients. Patients who take action, change their lifestyles and add the right herbs and vitamins to their diets really can achieve a lot towards managing their symptoms!

The second lesson is that she didn't give up on finding a solution to her cognitive issues when her first treatment option didn't work as well as she wanted. Too often, patients try something that doesn't work for them, and then give up or assume that their health care provider can't help them. This is so unfortunate! I talk a lot about individualizing therapy to meet your needs. Often times, this will take more than one try to get it exactly right for you. **Don't give up if your first option isn't everything you had hoped for! There are many worthwhile options to consider!**

The third lesson to take away from Christine's story is that she kept an open dialogue with her menopause provider. She was honest about what was working and what wasn't. She was curious and asked questions about medicinal and hormonal therapies. In today's healthcare environment, staying involved and connected are very important. Your menopause advisor can help with suggestions and information, however a successful outcome is ultimately a result of an open-minded partnership between you and your provider.

And finally, it is worth noting that patients like Christine, who require hormone therapies, belong to a small portion of my patients, but they are still a part of my practice. Many of my patients are able to manage their symptoms very well using only natural therapies and lifestyle changes. Some will require a medicinal or hormonal therapy to achieve optimal relief. No matter where you fall in this spectrum, you can and should expect safe and effective relief of your symptoms.

As discussed in Chapter 5, I categorize therapies into three broad areas:

- Natural therapies
- Medicinal therapies
- Hormone therapies

Within each of these categories there are numerous options that have proven beneficial in the treatment of specific and/or multiple symptoms associated with menopause. As I've mentioned, you must use the right doses, in the right combinations, and for the right period of time to maximize your benefit from any of the options I discuss here. The rest of this chapter will be devoted to providing information on each of the specific recommended options within each of these three categories.

NATURAL THERAPIES

1. Lifestyle Changes

Lifestyle changes are the hallmark of natural therapies, but are perhaps the most difficult to implement as they do require changes in how we go about our day. It is well documented in the literature that they work, and I see successes with my patients every day. Strategies many patients use to successfully manage their menopause symptoms include:

- **Stay Cool:** Based on the known mechanisms of hot flashes and night sweats, it's not surprising that just staying cool works for many women. Lower the thermostat, use fans (especially overhead fans), and turn up the air conditioner if necessary. Keep a folding fan in your purse for those times you can't directly control your environment. Sip iced drinks, preferably water or juice, at the start of a hot flash. Dress in layers so that you can remove one layer at a time if you get warm. Use light sheets and clothing that lets your skin breath, such as cotton or linen, rather than synthetic fabrics such as nylon, polyester or rayon. The Sharper Image makes a neck cooling device ($39.00) that has a small battery operated fan which blows cooled water through the necklace, cooling your upper body in really warm weather. All of these methods can help keep your hot flashes at bay.

- **Learn Deep Breathing Techniques:** Because adrenaline is involved, deep breathing techniques and other methods of relaxation such as meditation and hypnosis can help many menopausal symptoms, including hot flashes, night sweats, mood changes, sleep disruption and cognitive symptoms. Pranayama is the breathing technique used in yoga, which may be a great place to start as you'll get exercise, too!

- **Stop Smoking:** You may feel like menopause, with the stress of the symptoms, is not the time to try and quit. Actually, any time is a good time, and menopause is definitely a time that you'll feel immediate benefits from quitting! The medical literature is clear that smoking makes most menopause symptoms worse. Smoking increases the body's metabolism of estrogen, making estrogen levels even lower in smokers than in non-smokers. Due to the lowered level of estrogen, smokers tend to experience menopause symptoms, on average, two years sooner than in non-smokers. There are many strategies you can employ to try and quit, and there are many books, web pages, and organizations dedicated to smoking cessation, so I'm not going to spend a lot of time discussing ways to quit. I do recommend looking at the American Lung Association's website at www.lungusa.org and going through the wealth of information they have gathered on the effects of smoking in women, smoking cessation, and their online action plan that will help you individualize your journey to being smoke-free. (If you can't stop without taking medications, the new medicine Chantix® has worked in many of our patients.) Quitting smoking now will not only reduce your hot flashes and night sweats, but will reduce your risk for a wide variety of chronic diseases. Don't wait any longer to quit smoking! Take action today!

- **Make Dietary Changes:** Spicy foods, alcohol, and caffeine can trigger hot flashes in some women. Many patients tell us that a glass of wine at dinner will often lead to significant night sweats later that night. Test yourself. If these substances cause symptoms, make appropriate changes. If you just can't live without your morning coffee or your salsa fix, then make a point of keeping hydrated and always drink plenty of fluids.

- **Lose Weight:** Women who are overweight have more hot flashes than women who aren't. Researchers suspect this is because body fat acts as insulation, keeping women hotter. Losing weight, then, becomes an important way to reduce your hot flashes and other symptoms! Simple measures can help you lose weight, and losing weight has benefits beyond just reducing menopausal symptoms. BMI (body mass index) and weight loss strategies are discussed further in Chapter 7.

- **Exercise Regularly and Effectively:** Numerous studies have shown that exercise, in addition to having multiple health benefits, reduces hot flashes, night sweats and changes in mood and cognition. If you don't already do it, beginning an exercise program right away should be an important part of your plan for management of your menopause. You definitely want to discuss your exercise regimen with your healthcare professional to help maximize your benefits and reach reasonable goals. Remember that simple measures can make a big difference in the long term! More on what kinds and how much exercise I suggest can be found in Chapter 7.

2. Herbs, Vitamins, and Natural Supplements

Many of my patients use herbs, vitamins, and other natural substances successfully for relieving hot flashes, night sweats, mood changes, and cognitive deficiencies. However, there are so many natural substances being marketed, and so many studies on them reporting conflicting outcomes, that physicians as well as patients are left wondering what really works. Unfortunately, friends and heath food store clerks making recommendations is not a safe way to manage your health care, as some of these substances can cause adverse and/or unintended effects.

To make matters worse, some brands of herbs are less effective or less trustworthy regarding purity than other brands. No wonder this area is so confusing! Don't let friends, health food store clerks, or the Internet be your doctor. **I am here to help you cut through the confusion and develop a plan that you can feel confident to follow.**

There are many herbs that you will commonly see recommended for menopause symptoms. **For many of these common herbs, there is enough controversy about their effectiveness or concern over their safety and/or purity that we do not recommend that you start with just any of these supplements.**

Rather, let me make it simple for you by recommending a combination of a few vitamins and herbs known to be effective and safe for most women at menopause. I have recommended this combination that I call **"The Perfect Menopause Natural Therapy Formula"** for many years, and my patients have enjoyed significant success in reducing their symptoms.

"THE PERFECT MENOPAUSE NATURAL THERAPY FORMULA"

- **One multivitamin per day:** A multivitamin contains a balance of supplemental vitamins and nutrients necessary for good health, which may be lacking in contemporary diets. In addition to their own specific benefits, these vitamins act in concert with the other supplements listed below to optimize the management of symptoms. It is generally not necessary to buy an expensive multivitamin. There are good, inexpensive, multivitamins on the market. For example, a generic version of Centrum or One-A-Day vitamins are good choices. Use the regular multivitamin if you are in the perimenopause, or the "Silver" formulation if you are in menopause. The major difference between the two formulations is that the regular multivitamin contains extra iron. You won't need the extra iron when you are finished with your periods. Extra iron will only cause stomach and intestinal irritation.

- **Vitamin E—400 to 1200 international units per day in addition to your multivitamin:** Vitamin E is recognized to help decrease hot flashes, night sweats, and brain fog. It also helps reduce breast tenderness, which is common during perimenopause and menopause. In addition, it acts synergistically with other herbs to increase their effectiveness. Begin with 400 International Units per day, and increase to 800 International Units, or 1200 International Units per day over the next three months, as needed, to reduce your symptoms. If you are on blood thinners or tend to bleed easily, discuss this first with your menopause advisor.

- **Fish Oils—1000 mg twice a day:** Fish oils contain omega–3 fatty acids in high concentration, and are helpful in maintaining low cholesterol levels and general cardiovascular health. Fish oils work to ease menopausal symptoms including hot flashes, night sweats, decreased mood swings, and brain fog. They also help with inflammatory processes, reducing fatigue and body aches as well as help maintain lower cholesterol levels. Some people find that fish oils upset their stomach. In that case, flaxseed oil may be substituted.

- **Black Cohosh—20 to 80 mg twice daily:** The literature supports black cohosh as the most successful herbal product in the treatment of hot flashes and night sweats. I have recommended this herb in the management of many patients over the course of many years, and I agree with the literature. Generally, it is safe and effective. In conjunction with the other herbs and vitamins listed here, it is even more effective.

  Start with 20 mg twice a day, and then increase to 40 mg twice a day after two weeks if you are still having symptoms. Most of our patients find that 40 mg twice a day is enough. If not, increase to 80 mg twice a day after four more weeks. Then, be patient and give it several weeks to work.

  Be aware—not all black cohosh preparations contain the actual ingredients. Recent laboratory assays of different supplements claiming to be black cohosh have confirmed this, and this has helped explain why some patients do not respond as expected. Remifemin® is the most respected and most studied of the brand-label black cohosh preparations available. We strongly recommend that you stick to this brand. Remember, too, that anything you take has potential side effects. Just because it is a plant product does not automatically make it safe. We use black cohosh a great deal in our practice, but make sure your doctor(s) feel(s) it is right for you.

WARNING! There is some recent literature suggesting that black cohosh has the potential to cause liver toxicity in certain patients. As I write, there is an ongoing debate over this. In some European countries, warning labels have been put on black cohosh. To be safe, don't take this herb if you have liver problems, yellow skin, or serious medical problems. Talk to a qualified provider first. And I strongly suggest liver function testing (blood tests) before starting black cohosh, as well as routine follow-up tests of liver function while taking this herb. Black cohosh also interferes with anticoagulants. Don't take it if you are on anticoagulants or have a bleeding disorder.

- **Red Clover Leaf—One 40-mg tablet per day:** Red clover leaf is an alternative to black cohosh. Very similar in its mechanism of action and result, I often use this herb when there is concern about black cohosh. Promensil® is a popular brand. If you are concerned about using black cohosh because of the liver toxicity issue, use red clover leaf as the alternative. Although there aren't the same liver toxicity concerns with red clover leaf as there are with black cohosh, be sure to discuss red clover leaf with your provider before you begin taking this herb.

- **St. John's Wort—300 mg three times a day:** A very popular herb, St. John's wort is very effective in the treatment of mild-to-moderate depression and mood changes. When used in combination with black cohosh (or red clover leaf), these two herbs have a synergistic effect on each other, and symptoms such as hot flashes, night sweats and mood changes are improved. St. John's wort is safe and effective, but it can interfere with some other medicines such as the birth control pill. It may also cause some increased photosensitivity, so use an appropriate sun block and a hat. Most popular brands are acceptable, such as Nature's Way or Centrum. Don't take St. John's wort if you are taking Prozac, Zoloft, or any of the SSRI antidepressant medications. And be sure to take it at the correct dose three times per day.

- **Gingko Biloba—120 mg two times a day:** Designated as the "herb of the decade" a few years ago, Gingko biloba is a very popular and effective herb. It is thought to improve blood flow and is effective in improving intermittent claudication, a condition that causes leg cramps. It is also useful for improved cognition, including concentration, focus and memory. Gingko biloba has also been used for improving libido and orgasms by increasing blood flow to the genitals. For improvement with sexual performance, an additional dose of 120 mg an hour or so before intimacy is recommended.

- **Ginseng—I Prefer Siberian Ginseng (Siberian Eleuthero)—500 mg two or even three times a day**: Ginseng is one of the most effective herbs for many uses. For menopause, it helps reduce the symptoms of hot flashes, night sweats and mood dysfunction. It is also known to increase both emotional and physical energy. Ginseng boosts metabolism, which may help you keep your weight down. It may also improve the immune system. Believe it or not, ginseng is also known to increase sex drive. Start with one capsule a day, and increase to two or three capsules. Too much ginseng may make you feel jittery, as though you had too much coffee. Do not take after dinner as ginseng may make you restless at night.

Another option if you cannot find Siberian ginseng (and it can be hard to find sometimes) is Korean or Panex ginseng, 500 mg once or twice a day.

- **Maca—2,000-3,000 mg one time per day:** Maca may be an alternative to ginseng. It is sometimes called Peruvian ginseng, although it is not a ginseng per se. It is very effective for hot flashes, night sweats, energy and sexual dysfunction. Take Maca or ginseng, or both.

HOW TO USE "THE PERFECT MENOPAUSE" NATURAL SUPPLEMENT FORMULA

Start with one supplement and after two or three days, add the next. By two weeks, you will be taking the entire formula. (See Figure 6–1.) Give everything three months to work. Herbs and other natural therapies take time! They are milder than traditional medicines, and you will not notice an effect initially. Don't give up too soon. And take them regularly!

Figure 6–1
"The Perfect Menopause Natural Supplement Formula" Dosing Schedule

Start Day	Supplement or Herb	Dosage
Day 1	Multivitamin	1 pill, once per day
Day 3	Vitamin E	400 IU, 1–3 times per day
Day 5	Fish Oils	1,000 mg, 2 times per day
Day 7	Black Cohosh —or— Red Clover Leaf	20–80 mg, 2 times per day 40 mg, once per day
Day 9	St. John's Wort	300 mg, 3 times per day
Day 11	Gingko Biloba	120 mg, 2 times per day
Day 13	Siberian Ginsing —or— Maca	500 mg, 1–3 times per day 2000-3000 mg once per day

WHAT ABOUT OTHER SUPPLEMENTS?

Are you taking another supplement that is working for you? If you have a different supplement that is working for you, then I recommend that you continue to use it. I do recommend that you check it out with your menopause provider to make sure it is safe and does not contain any worrisome ingredients. I also recommend that you consult your physician before adding any new herbs to ensure that you won't have any side effects due to taking multiple substances together.

SOME HERBS SIMPLY DON'T WORK FOR MENOPAUSE; OTHERS HAVE SERIOUS SIDE EFFECTS

Based on many years of experience, as well as evaluation of the literature, I have found that soy products and evening primrose oil alone are just not as effective in reducing symptoms as the formula I recommend. Soy products and evening primrose oil are great products in general, and I believe both have some health benefits. Soy products are generally healthy, and evening primrose oil is a rich source of omega–3 fatty acids, which can also be very useful for the management of breast tenderness. There will always be exceptions, and I do recommend these substances in certain circumstances. However I suggest you start with my formula first.

Make Sure Your Herbs Don't Interact with Your Other Medicines. Talk to your qualified medical provider—one who is knowledgeable about your medicines and your herbs. And make sure your herbs and natural therapies won't adversely interact with your other medicines.

Consult ConsumerLab.com. For any brand of herbs other than those mentioned in this book, I strongly recommend that you check ConsumerLab.com for their purity, safety, and content before buying or using them. This is imperative if you want to guarantee the best possible results from your herbal therapy!

IMPORTANT: I can only recommend what I see works for my patients, but I do not have access to your medical history and can't tell you if everything I recommend is absolutely safe for you to take or not!

Before you start taking any herbs, vitamins, or other natural substances, be sure to discuss them with your menopause expert.

Massage Therapy, Acupuncture, Meditation, Hypnosis, Yoga, Pilates, Tae Chi, and Qigong

Massage therapy, acupuncture, meditation, hypnosis, yoga, Pilates, Tae Chi, and Qigong, are all effective means of relieving many of the symptoms of menopause, and indeed very helpful for many other health issues, too. Known as mind/body treatments, these therapies are based on eastern medicine practices and center on focusing the body's energy to heal. There are numerous health benefits in each of the treatments. I highly recommend these powerful therapies, and I have many patients who pursue these therapies. I myself practice meditation, hypnosis, and Qigong with numerous health benefits, and find them so helpful that I have trained to teach them.

These modalities all take time, and they must be practiced regularly. But if you pursue them regularly, they will reward you with many health benefits, including help with your menopause symptoms. There are excellent CDs and books in major bookstores on these disciplines, and several are listed in Chapter 13. Get a good resource or take a class. You will be impressed.

Medicinal Therapies

When natural therapies don't work for your major symptoms, medicinal or hormonal therapies ought to be considered. Hormone therapies may not be appropriate for some patients who are at an elevated risk for, or who have already had, estrogen-dependent breast or uterine cancer. For these patients, medicinal therapies may be extremely useful.

Since the early 1900s, there have been attempts to use many different medicines to treat the hot flashes, night sweats and mood changes that are associated with the menopause. For some women, they work better than herbal and other natural therapies. However, each medicine has potential side effects, and medicines may not be as effective as hormone therapies in improving the symptoms that you are seeking to alleviate.

Older medications such as Bellergal® alkaloids, the anti-hypertensive Clonidine, Lofexidine or Aldomet®, and the dopamine antagonist Veralipride, have been tried for the reduction of hot flashes and night sweats. However, they are only minimally effective and have a high side effect profile.

More recently, however, newer medicinal therapies have been used with greater success. The anti-seizure medicine Neurontin® (gabapentin), or the mild antidepressants and mood stabilizers (known as SSRIs) such as Effexor®, Paxil®, Prozac®, and Zoloft® have been found to have some effectiveness for relieving hot flashes, night sweats and mood dysfunction. Some individuals experience side effects, but these medicines may be worth trying if you have considerable symptoms. Some of my patients are being treated with these agents and feel much better. If you choose to pursue medicinal therapy, I recommend the following options:

- **Consider one of the SSRIs first:** In my patients, Effexor at a very low dose provides the best balance between efficacy and side effects. Start with 37.5 mg per day, and this will likely be enough. This low dose may also keep side effects to a minimum. If your symptoms do not improve after several weeks, increase the dose to 75 mg per day. Side effects of all of the SSRIs in some women may include sexual dysfunction (decreased libido and/or orgasmic ability), fatigue, dry mouth, constipation, nausea, and weight gain. One pharmaceutical company is researching a refined Effexor (called Pristiq™) for these symptoms. Low doses of some other SSRIs may also work (Paxil at 12.5 to 25 mg per day, Prozac at 10 to 20 mg per day, and Zoloft at 25 to 50 mg per day). In my patient population, those on Paxil, in particular, tend to gain weight.

  In my experience, approximately two-thirds of my patients taking SSRIs reduced their hot flashes, night sweats, and mood changes by at least 50%. Sexual dysfunction is the most common side effect in my patients. If you have sexual symptoms before beginning a medicine, try Neurontin first.

- **Neurontin (also known as Gabapentin):** If the SSRIs do not work or produce unacceptable side effects, try Neurontin. Neurontin is a well-known, mild, anti-seizure medication which is also often used for chronic pain syndromes. Recent research has discovered that it is also useful for treating hot flashes and night sweats. It does not help much with mood swings or cognitive deficiencies such as memory or fuzzy focus, but it may help with body aches and pains. In my practice, two-thirds of my patients taking Neurontin find that it reduces the hot flashes and night sweats by approximately 50%. Potential side effects include dizziness and fatigue. Start with 300 mg a day in the morning. After 3 days add a second 300 mg dose in the evening. After another 3 days, add a third 300 mg dose at noon, for a total of 900 mg per day. This is the most commonly effective dose, however some patients require much higher doses, even up to twice this amount (1800 mg/day).

Please note that there are many other medicinal therapies that are available to treat specific symptoms, such as sleep disturbance and sexual dysfunction, associated with the menopause. We will be addressing those symptoms and treatments in subsequent chapters. The medicines discussed here in Chapter 6 are those that have been shown to have the most usefulness in treating hot flashes, night sweats, mood changes, and in some cases, cognitive issues, and muscle or joint pain.

HORMONE THERAPIES

If natural therapies and medicinal therapies don't work or are not appealing to you, consider hormone therapies. **Hormone therapies are the most effective of all the therapies for the treatment of symptoms associated with the menopause.**

If you are against hormone therapies, please don't stop reading yet. Find out for yourself what this is all about. Don't get lost in the emotion. Many new patients come to see me each week with several preconceived notions that are incorrect, and a significant misunderstanding of hormone therapies. **Don't forget, "The answers have changed."** If hormone therapy has become an option for you, consider the facts—not the media's latest take, your neighbor's experience, and so on. Would you let your neighbor tell you which blood pressure medicine to take? Consider all the latest facts. The latest information on the hormone studies, as well as assessments of the benefits, risks, advantages and disadvantages of hormone therapies, are presented in Chapters 2, 3 and 5. Use the information in those chapters as well as this one to properly assess whether hormone therapy may be right for you.

WHEN APPROPRIATE, HORMONE THERAPIES MAY MAKE A TREMENDOUS DIFFERENCE IN HOW YOU FEEL, AND MAY IMPROVE YOUR HEALTH IN GENERAL

If you decide to use a hormone therapy, there are numerous estrogens, progestogens, and combinations available. **They are not all the same**. In fact, hormones are available in a wide variety of preparations. Variations on hormone preparations include a variety of estrogen molecules (micronized, conjugated, bioidentical), dosage strength, delivery system (oral transdermal, etc.), systemic preparations (designed to work throughout your system via your bloodstream), and local preparations (designed to help certain tissues with minimal absorption into the bloodstream). Based on the latest research and my many years of practical patient management, I recommend that you consider the following guidelines for the safest and best outcomes:

1. Have A Complete Medical Evaluation First: This includes a complete physical exam and baseline blood tests (blood count, metabolic profile, liver function tests, glucose and lipid profile). Also, I recommend a complete baseline hormonal evaluation, including blood levels of estradiol, estrone, serum free testosterone, DHEA sulfate, and thyroid levels. A baseline mammogram and the DEXA bone density test is also recommended. Depending on your age and family history, a colonoscopy and electrocardiogram should also be considered.

2. Try the Transdermal Estrogens First: I recommend starting with a transdermal patch. Unlike oral estrogen, transdermal estrogen does not go through the liver on its first pass through the body. Therefore, the clotting factors that are produced as a byproduct of oral estrogen making its first pass in the liver are minimally affected. This eliminates the slight increase in risk of blood clots and strokes that is seen with oral estrogens.

Although I have several patients who use the transdermal estrogen gels and creams successfully, the patches are effective, convenient, and have the benefits of exact dosing and consistent transmission of estrogen through the skin. Patches also eliminate the accidental transmission of hormones to people in contact with you, a phenomenon which has been reported with patients using creams and gels. If you would prefer transdermal creams or gels, they are generally effective and you should work with your menopause provider to determine which option is best for you.

3. Use the Lowest Effective Dose: There are many doses of transdermal patches available, and for all creams and gels, a dose can be tailored to your individual needs. Start with a very low dose, and increase slowly, if necessary, to a dose suitable for your symptoms. I am completely aware of the recently promoted Suzanne Somers' recommendation to use high doses of hormones at levels consistent with those when you were much younger. Please keep in mind that there is no scientific evidence to show benefits of these higher doses, and absolutely no scientific evidence to show the safety of this recommendation. **In fact, the best data to date would suggest that high doses are highly risky and potentially very harmful.**

4. Use Bioidentical Hormones If Possible: While there is absolutely no data to show that bioidentical hormones are better or safer, it makes absolute sense to me as a chemist, gynecologist, and natural therapist, that bioidentical hormones are theoretically better. I prefer using estradiol. It is the estrogen produced by the ovary. We understand its metabolism in the body, and can measure it, and its metabolites, in blood levels. For a more thorough discussion of bioidentical hormones, please refer back to Chapter 3.

Start with a 0.025 mg or a 0.0375 mg transdermal estradiol patch (or similar low dose of creams or gels which are available commercially or can be compounded and similarly used), and adjust up or down depending on your results. Many women complain that generic patches do not stick well and sometimes irritate the skin. If this is your experience, the brand-name patches (Climara® or Vivelle® Dot) may be better for you. The patches are usually placed on the lower abdomen near where the ovaries are.

If you prefer a compounded bioidentical product, I recommend the very popular Biest (see Chapter 3) skin cream which is often compounded with natural progesterone. Use 2.5 mg of Biest with 100 mg of progesterone. The cream is usually applied twice a day to the skin. I recommend the lower abdomen, arms, or thighs—not the chest area.

Compounding pharmacies can compound any bioidentical hormone or combination at any dose. If you prefer compounded, your menopause provider will help you with the choices.

Compounding pharmacies usually do not produce patches, but often sell the commercially available ones.

5. You May Also Need Progesterone: If you have had a hysterectomy, you may not need progesterone at all (although some of you with a hysterectomy might benefit from added progesterone). If you have not had a hysterectomy, you will need a small amount of progesterone periodically to protect the lining of your uterus. As with estrogen, I prefer the use of bioidentical progesterone. Unfortunately, it is not yet available as a transdermal patch, and progesterone transdermal creams and gels at low doses are not generally regarded as effective at protecting the lining of the uterus. Progesterone can be taken orally as micronized progesterone, or the same micronized progesterone pill can be absorbed by placing it into the vagina. Progesterone can also be used as a progesterone suppository or gel.

While progesterone may help with perimenopausal symptoms, progesterone alone usually does not help with symptoms as menopause progresses, and for many women it can cause a return to PMS symptoms. Therefore, I prefer to use it minimally. **To start, I use what is called the "long cycle," which is 12 days of bioidentical oral progesterone every 3 months.** The typical oral (or vaginal) dose is 200 mg and is available as either a compounded product or commercially as Prometrium®. Progesterone may produce a mild menstrual period in some women. **It may also make you sleepy, and I always recommend taking it at bedtime.** Vaginal progesterone creams or gels can also be compounded or is commercially available as a 4% vaginal cream (Prochieve® or Crinone®). When used in "long cycle" treatment, Prochieve or Crinone is dosed as one applicator every other night for a total of 7 doses, with this process repeated every three months. See Figure 6–2 for more details.

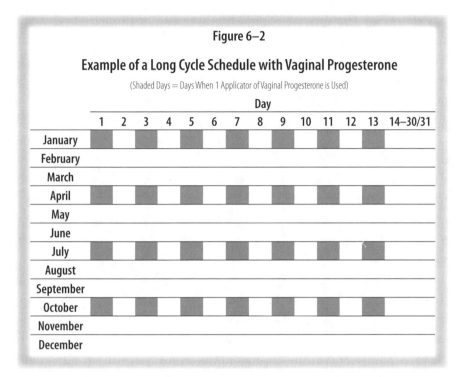

Figure 6–2

Example of a Long Cycle Schedule with Vaginal Progesterone

(Shaded Days = Days When 1 Applicator of Vaginal Progesterone is Used)

	Day													
	1	2	3	4	5	6	7	8	9	10	11	12	13	14–30/31
January	■		■		■		■			■		■		
February														
March														
April	■		■		■		■			■		■		
May														
June														
July	■		■		■		■			■		■		
August														
September														
October	■		■		■		■			■		■		
November														
December														

6. Monitor Your Therapy Closely with Your Menopause Provider: Check hormone levels, and correlate this measurement with how you are feeling. This will help you decide on the correct hormone levels, and will help you maintain optimal levels of hormones as you follow your therapy over time. Find the dose that is "right" for you as an individual.

7. Follow-up Breast Exams: Three months after you begin estrogen, follow up with your provider for a breast exam, and have a mammogram within the first six months. The re-analyses of the WHI showed that estrogen is NOT the likely cause of breast cancer, but it may accelerate blood flow to an existing tumor, causing the tumor to grow more quickly in size. Please note: a tumor growing in size is significantly different from a tumor spreading. A tumor that grows larger is more easily palpable (felt) or is more likely to be **visible on a mammogram sooner.** Some experts feel that using estrogen may actually be a benefit in the earlier detection of breast cancer due to the possibility of earlier detection of larger tumors. **It may even explain why, among breast cancer patients, those who used estrogen live longer than those who don't.**

8. Report Any Unexpected Vaginal Bleeding and be Properly Evaluated:
Unexpected vaginal bleeding is not normal at any time during menopause,
and could indicate hyperplasia or tumor growth (both cancerous and non-
malignant). Expected or scheduled bleeding is vaginal bleeding when you
take and/or finish the progesterone. Unexpected or unscheduled bleeding is
any time other than this. Notify your menopause provider of any unexpected
vaginal bleeding. It is important to have an evaluation to determine the cause
of this bleeding. Many gynecologists and menopause experts today use vaginal ultrasound with fluid (a sonohysterogram), an easy office evaluation, to
make this determination.

9. Vaginal Estrogen: If you are using the lowest possible dose of hormones
to treat hot flashes, night sweats, mood changes, and cognitive issues, it may
not be enough estrogen to treat for vaginal dryness and painful intercourse
from thin vaginal tissues. If this is the case for you, or if your only menopausal symptoms are localized to your vagina, then you should consider using
vaginal estrogens for your vaginal symptoms. The use of vaginal estrogens is
discussed in greater detail in Chapter 8. **The use of systemic estrogen is not
recommended for the sole purpose of vaginal dryness.**

10. Oral Estrogen: If you do not do well with transdermal estradiol patches,
creams or gels, or prefer oral therapies, estradiol (the bioidentical estrogen)
is available as an oral preparation. The bioidentical estradiol pill has a very
rapid gastrointestinal absorption. This means that it must be taken at least
twice a day in order to maintain a constant, therapeutically effective blood
level. Even then, variable levels are found in the bloodstream. Because of this,
higher doses of estrogen (as compared to oral plant derived conjugated estrogens or transdermal estrogens) often must be used in order to maintain the
estrogen levels in your bloodstream at therapeutic levels throughout the day.

  For a compounded oral hormone product, Biest is available (and very
popular) with or without progesterone.

  Use Biest 2.5 mg with 100 mg of progesterone per day, but dosed as a
twice a day product to maintain blood level.

  Another oral estrogen that I use in my practice is Estradiol acetate (Fem-
trace®), which is commercially available as an oral preparation. Estradiol

acetate is a chemically modified estradiol that absorbs more slowly over the day than "plain" estradiol. Once ingested, estradiol acetate is transformed by the liver into estradiol.

There are two excellent, commercially-available products that I prescribe that contain conjugated estrogens. A conjugated estrogen is an estrogen molecule that has a sulfate salt molecule attached to it in order to be absorbed. These "new technology" pills employ a specialized construction that allows the pills to dissolve slowly in layers, somewhat like the way a jawbreaker candy dissolves, which make once-a-day dosing possible. Enjuvia™ and Cenestin™ use plant-derived estrogens, but because of the attached salt molecule, and the mixture of estrogens, these estrogens are not completely bioidentical. When oral estrogens are considered, these products have an advantage of being able to be used effectively at extremely low doses. In these circumstances, they are a great choice for patients who prefer once-a-day oral therapy. **Individualization in hormone therapy is always preferred.**

11. Testosterone: What about testosterone? It is not likely that the average woman going through menopause will also be going through simultaneous andropause. Your testosterone level, while it should be measured, will likely be normal. If it is not, testosterone therapy should be initiated with bioidentical testosterone pills, creams, or gels. Testosterone products for women are currently only available through a compounding pharmacy. Appropriate doses of testosterone are further discussed in Chapter 9.

12. What About DHEA? DHEA can be an important hormone in the menopause and perimenopause time. Although the use of it in standard hormone therapy regimens is limited, on occasion, small amounts of DHEA supplementation makes sense and is useful. The most important current uses of DHEA is for impaired memory and cognition. The standard dose is usually 25 mg for women. But many articles in the literature show that much lower doses can be effective. Even 12.5 mg or less may be enough for the female.

In the body, DHEA breaks down into estrogen, testosterone, and other minor components. Therefore, when I treat a woman with DHEA, I also monitor her hormone levels. I follow blood levels of her estradiol, estrone, free testosterone, and DHEA sulfate.

Figure 6–3

"The Perfect Menopause" Hormone Therapy

- Begin with a low dose, bioidentical, transdermal estradiol product.
- Adjust up or down slightly depending on symptoms.
- Follow blood levels of estrogen (estradiol and estrone).
- Have a breast exam in three months and a mammogram in three to six months.
- Add bioidentical oral progesterone 200 mg (at bedtime) for 12 nights every three months (or equivalent vaginal progesterone).
- Use testosterone and/or DHEA when clinically appropriate.

WHY NOT USE PREMARIN® AND PREMPRO®?

There are several reasons why I don't use them. Premarin utilizes horse urine extraction technology developed in 1942, and due to this process, these products contain known impurities. Chemists in medicine, like me, are nervous about impurities. Additionally, the Provera® (the synthetic non-bioidentical progestin) contained in Prempro has been identified as the potential cause of some of the negative effects in the WHI 2002 study. With all the other modern hormone products on the market today for menopausal management which we know do not contain impurities, in my opinion, Premarin and Prempro just aren't the best, most up-to-date products available. Please refer back to Chapters 2 and 5 for a thorough discussion of Premarin and Prempro (Premarin plus the synthetic progestin Provera) if you would like more detail than what is presented here.

DON'T GET CONFUSED AND LOST IN EMOTIONS!

Making a decision on what therapies to take can be very difficult. Opinions abound. Ask around or search online if you need proof! Eventually, you have to trust someone to give you the best possible advice.

It takes a great deal of knowledge, tremendous perspective, and many years of practical experience to safely advise an individual patient about the best and safest management possible. Use the thoughts in this book as a way to gain perspective on your own situation, and use this knowledge to start a dialogue with your menopause provider.

Every treatment has its benefits as well as risks. While I'd prefer that my patients try natural therapies first, I also recognize that some of the natural therapies (even herbs and vitamins) can have side effects and unexpected consequences. If there are side effects, they are likely to be minor, but not always. Similarly, there are potential side effects for medicinal therapies. For hormone therapies, when they are the most appropriate option, I have outlined a very safe and effective approach to using them in the management of the menopause.

WHICH IS SAFER?

Which of these options is safest? Depending on your situation, I propose they all could be equally safe. Be open-minded, and remember that the answers have changed! There is considerable new data on all of these therapeutic options.

MANAGE MAJOR SYMPTOMS

In Step 2, you took a closer look at your menopausal symptoms and developed a set of goals for your therapy. In Step 3, you learned specifics about natural, medicinal, and hormonal therapies that I recommend for my patients to manage major symptoms, and why some of them work. Now that you've read this chapter, you can begin to make assessments of what type of therapies might be right for you based on your symptoms and their severity.

You may have discovered that some of the lifestyle changes that help alleviate hot flashes are the same lifestyle changes you've been meaning to make for years! Well, now is the time! Or, you might have discovered that even though you have a history of breast cancer in the family, you don't have to suffer through terrible hot flashes and can try a medicinal therapy. You might have even discovered that hormones may make sense for you to consider after all! I sincerely hope that whatever your conclusions, you have discovered that there are many safe and effective options for you to try. I also hope that you've gained a sense of how to navigate your way, with the help of your menopause provider, through the wide range of options available to you. **You can and will find something that works for you, I guarantee it**.

In the Natural Therapy section of this chapter, we briefly addressed weight loss as a lifestyle change that can help you alleviate symptoms. Some of you may want to just lose weight anyway, and feel like you've tried every way possible to get rid of those extra pounds that creeped up on you during menopause! In the next chapter, Step 4, I hope to help you "Get to Your Perfect Weight" with a few proven methods. You'll not only lose pounds, you will also help reduce your major menopausal symptoms and feel and look great doing it!

chapter

7

Step Four
Get To Your Perfect Weight

ARE YOU HAPPY WITH YOUR WEIGHT? Or have you noticed a few extra pounds have settled around your waist? Are you frustrated because you feel that you eat right and exercise, but you still manage to gain weight?

Maybe You Can Relate To Judy:

Judy is a 51 year old dietitian. At her annual gynecologic exam last year, she told me that she had gained 40 pounds in the last eight years. "I eat well, I exercise, and I still can't stop gaining," she said. We talked about nutrition and re-examined her eating and exercise habits. We discussed that she had gained an average of 5 pounds per year, and how the changes her body has been going through during perimenopause and menopause may be affecting her metabolism. Then, we developed a weight-loss plan.

When she returned for her exam this year, I couldn't believe my eyes. She looked wonderful and she gushed that, she "feels great!" She had lost the entire 40 pounds in one year! She said that her successful weight loss was made possible with the plan we worked out, plus the encouragement of our office staff.

Let's change your weight situation beginning today. In this chapter, you will learn the 7 steps to losing weight healthily, creating a slim waist, and feeling better about yourself!

WHAT CAUSES MIDLIFE WAIST EXPANSION?

Weight gain is the number one complaint of my patients. Menopause practitioners know that between the ages of 35 and 55 you will either gain weight or find that maintaining your weight becomes much more difficult. Also, weight gained at this time of your life will tend to accumulate around your waist, rather than your hips and thighs. Eventually you will notice an increase in weight in your face and neck, as well as in your breasts. Some women gain a substantial amount of weight during this period of life.

"MENOPOT"

Dr. Pamela Peeke, in her excellent book, *Body For Life For Women,* elaborates on the midlife waist expansion and describes the "menopot" as that compartment of menopausal belly fat accumulated outside the abdominal muscle. The good news is this is different from the more dangerous or "toxic" portion of the belly fat underneath the abdominal wall, around organs, deep in the belly. But if my patients are any example, then regardless of whether the belly fat is inside or outside the abdominal muscle, you probably aren't fond of it.

No matter where the belly fat resides, the increased waist size is the single measurement most correlated with disease, especially cardiovascular disease and death. A recent study from the University of Texas Southwestern Medical Center showed that weight alone did not predict the chances of early artery clogging, but that waistline size did. Simply put, they found that the smaller a person's waist, the clearer his or her arteries were observed to be.

WHAT DOES ESTROGEN HAVE TO DO WITH WEIGHT GAIN?

Doctors have known for a long time that the shifting levels of estrogen likely play a role in a metabolic change, causing subsequent weight gain. There is evidence to show that some women on estrogen therapy at menopause do have a slightly easier time controlling their weight and body shape. Fluctuating estrogen levels, however, only tell part of the story. Other causes of weight gain at midlife include:

- **Aging.** Aging itself leads to a decrease in metabolism and subsequent weight gain. As you age, your muscle mass decreases and your fat mass increases. One of my patients lamented that 10 years ago her body fat content was 27%. Today it is 37%. To make matters worse, as you gain weight your fat mass will increase even more. Because fat burns fewer calories than muscle, the reduced muscle and increased fat means that you will burn fewer calories for the same amount of exercise. All of this, of course, leads to even more weight increase.

- **Other hormone changes.** Balanced hormone levels are important in maintaining metabolism. Reduced levels of thyroid hormone are common in women around the menopause, and can lead to a decrease in metabolism and increase in weight. Progesterone and testosterone levels may also play a role in weight management. Estrogen levels decreasing at faster rates than testosterone levels (as in menopause) leads to a relative excess of testosterone, putting extra weight around the waist, chin, and neck.

- **Reduced physical activity**. Studies have shown that as we age, we tend to exercise less. Women at menopause usually exercise less than younger women, and reduced physical activity leads to weight gain.

- **Increased food intake**. Eating more means more calories taken in, which are converted to fat if you don't burn them through activity.

- **Genetics**. Your genes also play a role in weight gain. Scientists believe that some women are more predisposed to gain weight and change in shape. If you have this genetic predisposition, you may have to work harder to maintain a normal weight.

THE "HIDDEN IMPACT" OF WEIGHT GAIN

As your weight increases, you may dislike how you look, and you may not feel as healthy either. You will tend to feel more fatigued both physically and mentally. You will likely experience an increased shortness of breath. On top of all that, recent studies have shown that weight gain is associated with poorer sleep, and sleep is already a problem at menopause!

Weight gain can also increase your risk for heart disease. Those extra pounds make your cholesterol higher, your blood pressure higher, and your insulin resistance higher, which can lead to type 2 diabetes. Increased insulin resistance is also a risk factor for breast cancer. Clearly, the extra weight can be damaging not only to your self-image, but also to your long-term health and well-being.

TODAY'S FOODS AND EATING HABITS ARE A CONTRIBUTING FACTOR

We've known for a long time that there is a tendency to gain weight at menopause. However, in recent years, the magnitude of this weight gain has increased significantly. Your generation is gaining more weight at menopause than your mother's generation did. One of the reasons for this significant upward change has to do with the foods that are readily available to us.

DIRE PREDICTIONS

A recent study by scientists at Johns Hopkins University in Baltimore showed that 66% of U.S. adults are overweight or obese. Based on current trends, they project that number to be 75% by 2015.

Do these facts surprise you? Read further. Take action today. Don't let yourself be in this category!

Many of my patients feel that they eat healthily and exercise enough. They tell me that they are doing everything they can to lose weight, and that nothing is working. What I've discovered through the years, though, is that **most of us really do not know the elements of a healthy diet, even though we think we do.** Schools, even medical schools, do not adequately teach the concepts of nutrition and a healthy diet. Real knowledge about effective nutrition has changed also. Even the FDA's food pyramid changed in 2004! There are many current books that provide an overview of the latest knowledge about nutrition, so I won't go too deeply into the subject here. **What I want to impress upon you, though, is that most of us do not know the real, accurate, and up-to-date story of nutrition, and the medical profession's new understanding has not been effectively translated into practice. As Professor Einstein said, "The answers have changed."**

Trends in the way we eat have dramatically changed also, and not for the better. The documentary movie *Supersize Me* and the book *Fast Food Nation* expose some of the negative nutritional trends and their consequences. Today, we tend to eat foods high in simple carbohydrates and fats. Both of these challenge our body to produce insulin in larger amounts than usual. This results in transient (short-term) low blood sugar levels and feelings of hunger, which leads to more snacking, more insulin production, etc. This eating cycle leads to weight gain, frequent hunger, and the feeling that we can't get out of this cycle.

Even if we eat the servings recommended on the new food pyramid, the soils in which we grow our food have been increasingly depleted of essential nutrients. This means that these good foods are not packing the vitamins and minerals they once did, and we are not getting enough of these nutrients in a so-called proper diet. Additives and preservatives have significantly changed the health content of our foods, as well.

Many things have changed about food, and we simply haven't taken these changes into account as we consider good nutrition, our health, and weight management.

HOW WE EAT HAS CHANGED

Do you skip breakfast, or eat an inadequate one? Are the meals you do eat oversized? Do you eat too fast, or chew improperly? Do you drink enough fluids throughout the day and at meals? All these variables will also affect your metabolism.

Perhaps our "fast food society" has led to us eating faster and on the run, chewing less, skipping important meals (like breakfast), snacking more between meals, eating huge meals, and drinking less water. The expectation that everything can and should be done quickly has led to a few other "quick fix" eating behaviors that aren't healthy for us either.

CRASH DIETS

Most of us have tried at least one crash diet. Crash diets simply do not work. They may produce an initial positive result, but almost invariably there is a rebound weight gain. Your overall weight gain is often even more than your weight was to begin with! And crash diets are unhealthy! You can't possibly expect to get all the nutrients your body needs to maintain a healthy metabolism by eating, for example, nothing but pasta or grapefruit!

DO DIET PILLS REALLY DO THE JOB?
MORE BAD NEWS

Many patients look for pills or supplements to help them lose weight. And there is no shortage of products on the market claiming to help you in this endeavor. **Unfortunately, there is nothing available today that is considered safe, healthy, and effective**. All of those "weight loss" supplements come with considerable potential risks. You may remember that weight loss products which contained ephedrine were recently removed from the shelves after considerable side effects, including deaths, were reported. Pharmaceutical medicines which reduce food absorption also reduce absorption of some very essential nutrients, and this may be detrimental to your overall health. These so-called "remedies" are not the way to manage menopause weight gain!

BIG ADS INFLUENCE US

Big ads influence us because who among us doesn't want to find the easy way out with a magic pill or remedy? There continue to be numerous advertisements for supplements and herbs to curb your appetite or rev up your metabolism and help you lose weight.

There is much written on this subject by reputable natural medical therapists, and the world's experts in natural medicine will tell you that there simply is nothing safe and effective that you can "take" for weight loss.

WHAT ABOUT SURGERY?

Although there are risks to it, new laparoscopic techniques have made bariatric surgery a reasonable consideration for the extremely obese person. Surgery should only be considered for women with extreme obesity, for those who have been unable to lose weight by any other method, and for whom there will be medical consequences if they continue to fail to lose weight. These surgical procedures should be considered only after careful discussion with your entire health care team.

THE GOOD NEWS: YOU CAN CHANGE THIS SITUATION, BEGINNING TODAY!

The good news is you can lose weight, change your body shape for the better, and live healthier, happier, and with more energy. Plus you'll get the benefit of a significantly improved perimenopause and menopause! Having treated menopausal patients for over 25 years, I have seen and believe that you can and will manage your weight if you have a plan, an understanding of the plan and mechanisms, **and are willing to commit to this challenge.** Most patients who change their eating habits and start to exercise, have great success with losing weight. The changes I recommend will not only help you lose weight and keep it off, but will also likely lead to an improvement in the overall nutrition and health of both you and your loved ones, too. Everyone wins!

YOUR COMMITMENT, YOUR PLAN, AND YOUR COACH

The three elements for successful and lasting weight loss and body reconfiguration are:

- A plan that works,
- Commitment to the plan, and
- A coach to keep you on the course.

I am going to give you a plan, and with your menopause provider, I will be your coach. You must supply the commitment! **Are you ready for this commitment?** If you are ready to make a change, will commit to your plan, and believe that success can be achieved, **I guarantee that if you follow these 7 steps, you will lose weight, look and feel better, be healthier, and will have a significantly improved menopause.**

The Perfect Menopause Weight Loss Plan—7 Steps

There are seven steps to the perfect menopause weight loss plan:

1. Commit! And start today.
2. Establish your current profile, and then set your goals.
3. Measure your progress. Write it down in your journal.
4. Choose the right nutritional plan—low-carb versus low-fat.
5. Measure your portion size.
6. Choose your exercise plan.
7. Take action!

They sound simple enough, right? Again, though, it is not enough to just read this list! You've got to go through each step to reap the benefits. Let's discuss each step in more detail:

STEP 1: COMMIT! AND START TODAY

The first and most important step you can take is to commit to take action. You either want to change or you don't. Any good psychologist, coach, or personal motivator will tell you that you have to commit to change if there is going to be change. If you are serious about making a change, you will commit to take action. **Commit today, not tomorrow.** This is a basic and fundamental principle of making a change in your weight and body shape at perimenopause and menopause. There are no excuses here.

STEP 2: ESTABLISH YOUR CURRENT PROFILE, AND THEN SET YOUR GOALS

You must set specific goals if you are going to expect to be successful. This is probably the second hardest step of the weight-loss process, since setting goals now makes you accountable to your goals. But it is the only way you will achieve what you want! If we didn't shoot for the moon, Neil Armstrong never would have gotten to the moon! If you don't set an end goal with milestones to achieve along the way, then how do you expect to know if you are losing weight and changing your body shape or not?

In order to set your goal, you need to establish where you are now. Are you 10 pounds overweight? 20? 30? 50? 100? Where are you right now? Weigh yourself today. Look at yourself in the mirror and decide *what you want to change*. Get your true weight, height, and waist measurements. Write all of these measurements down in your progress journal, provided for you at the end of this chapter. Using those measurements, establish your Body Mass Index.

Calculate Your BMI

The Body Mass Index (BMI), was established in 1998 by the National Institute of Health, is a measure of body fat based on height and weight. The BMI system was used to learn about a patient's body composition in order to build a reference for what is considered normal and abnormal body composition, and to correlate the associated health risks. Based on your BMI, your menopause provider can help you make appropriate recommendations for improvement. Figure 7–1 will help you calculate your BMI from your height and weight. (Note: Measure your height without shoes. Don't guess).

Figure 7–1
Calculate Your Body Mass Index Table (BMI)

BMI	Normal 19	20	21	22	23	24	Overweight 25	26	27	28	29	Obese 30	31	32	33	34	35	36	37	38	39
Height (inches)	Body Weight (pounds)																				
58	91	96	100	105	110	115	119	124	129	134	138	143	148	153	158	162	167	172	177	181	186
59	94	99	104	109	114	119	124	128	133	138	143	148	153	158	163	168	173	178	183	188	193
60	97	102	107	112	118	123	128	133	138	143	148	153	158	163	168	174	179	184	189	194	199
61	100	106	111	116	122	127	132	137	143	148	153	158	164	169	174	180	185	190	195	201	206
62	104	109	115	120	126	131	136	142	147	153	158	164	169	175	180	186	191	196	202	207	213
63	107	113	118	124	130	135	141	146	152	158	163	169	175	180	186	191	197	203	208	214	220
64	110	116	122	128	134	140	145	151	157	163	169	174	180	186	192	197	204	209	215	221	227
65	114	120	126	132	138	144	150	156	162	168	174	180	186	192	198	204	210	216	222	228	234
66	118	124	130	136	142	148	155	161	167	173	179	186	192	198	204	210	216	223	229	235	241
67	121	127	134	140	146	153	159	166	172	178	185	191	198	204	211	217	223	230	236	242	249
68	125	131	138	144	151	158	164	171	177	184	190	197	203	210	216	223	230	236	243	249	256
69	128	135	142	149	155	162	169	176	182	189	196	203	209	216	223	230	236	243	250	257	263
70	132	139	146	153	160	167	174	181	188	195	202	209	216	222	229	236	243	250	257	264	271
71	136	143	150	157	165	172	179	186	193	200	208	215	222	229	236	243	250	257	265	272	279
72	140	147	154	162	169	177	184	191	199	206	213	221	228	235	242	250	258	265	272	279	287
73	144	151	159	166	174	182	189	197	204	212	219	227	235	242	250	257	265	272	280	288	295
74	148	155	163	171	179	186	194	202	210	218	225	233	241	249	256	264	272	280	287	295	303
75	152	160	168	176	184	192	200	208	216	224	232	240	248	256	264	272	279	287	295	303	311
76	156	164	172	180	189	197	205	213	221	230	238	246	254	263	271	279	287	295	304	312	320

For most adults, a BMI of less than 18.5 suggests that the person is underweight. A BMI between 18.5 and 24.9 is regarded as healthy and normal. A BMI between 24.9 and 29.9 is an indication of being overweight. BMI values of 30+ are categorized as obese. These categories are differentiated by the shading in Figure 7–1. Use Figure 7–1 to calculate your BMI, and record it in your progress journal as your baseline.

Establish Your Body Measurements

Now, measure your blood pressure, and all your body measurements (Figure 7–2). Take a photograph of yourself so that you may have a fair starting point from which to measure your progress. Put all of this information in your journal, too.

Figure 7–2

Body Measurements

Using a tape measure, measure your body measurements as follows:

Breasts:	Across your breasts:
Waist:	Across your waist at your belly button:
Menopot:	Across widest part of your abdomen:
Buttocks:	Across the widest part of your buttocks:
Arm:	Across the widest part of your upper arm:

Where Do You Want to Be?

Once you have established where you are today, close your eyes for a minute and decide where you would like your weight and body shape to be in 6 months, and then 12 months. Visualizing how you will look and feel will help you begin to establish your goals. See yourself stepping onto your scale, and watch it register the weight you wish to be. Think of yourself as that weight once again. (Some women even paste their idealized weight onto their scale, as further encouragement.) Write all of this down in your progress journal. Write down how you think you will feel when you reach your target weight, how you will look, and how your friends and family will react to this slimmer, trimmer, you.

Another Visualization Tool

John Abdo and Kenneth Dackman in their book, *Body Engineering*, suggest the following visualization for projecting your **new body image**. Stand before a full length mirror and get as naked as you can. Exhale while flexing your muscles. Then inhale, tighten your abdominals and stand up straight. This visualization exercise will help you in establishing a reasonable intermediate goal.

Use these visualization tools to help you achieve your goals. These are well-known exercises for the mind that help make your goal a reality. (Perhaps you'll recall Olympic athletes talking in interviews about using these very techniques before their events.) Visualize how you might look when you are at a smaller dress size, and then when you are fitting into the dress size you would like to be. Picture yourself going into an upscale store and choosing a new dress in your new size, or fitting into a trim pair of jeans. Or think about how it would feel to jog for 3 miles without wanting to collapse. Any one of these visualizations and goals will help you get to where you want to be with your weight and body shape. And keep your positive visualizations active every day.

You can reach any goal if you really want it and are willing to do what it takes to get there. When patients tell me that no matter what they do, they can't lose weight, I challenge them that weight loss is not important enough to them yet. When it becomes important enough, they will do whatever it takes and costs to reach their goal. Are you there yet? Use visualization and your imagination to come up with some goals that are really important to you. I strongly recommend that you set specific, yet realistic, goals. It is realistic and very helpful to set a 3-month, as well as a 6-, 9-, and 12-month goal right at the beginning.

From Goals to Action

Once you have established your goals, you'll need to work with your health care team to assess your medical situation. You may have already gotten a complete physical exam as part of your overall menopausal health management. If not, then call today to begin to work with your physician to establish your lipid profile, including your cholesterol, triglycerides, good cholesterol (HDL cholesterol), and bad cholesterol (LDL cholesterol). Also have your thyroid levels, blood count (hematocrit) and fasting glucose level measured. These values, if abnormal, may be relevant to your weight and body composition and have an impact on your weight loss programs. Record the results of these tests in your perfect menopause weight loss journal. You will be able to follow improvements in these values as you lose weight and restructure your body configuration.

Step 3: Measure Your Progress Write It Down In Your Journal

What you don't write down you won't remember, so it is very important that you keep a record of your progress. **When you write down your goals, and your progress toward them, your commitment becomes stronger!** As with the stock market, it is difficult to judge long-term changes based on the information available from a single day. In order to see a trend, you must have information over many days so that you can see that each little change is adding up. Losing half of an inch around your waist in 2 weeks may not seem like much, but do that every 2 weeks and in 2 months and you've dropped a dress size! Following your progress will help keep you inspired and motivated. Journaling is a well-known technique for success in achieving pre-determined goals. **Start today.**

Start by completing the first page of the perfect menopause weight loss program journal that is provided for you at the end of this chapter. Make copies of the second page, start your notebook, and keep exact records of your progress. **If you are not willing to commit to writing down your goals and progress, you are not determined enough yet to lose weight.** You can achieve any goal you set your mind to, but you have to be willing to do what it takes.

Have you seen the reality TV shows *The Biggest Loser* or *Celebrity Fit Club*? I think you would agree they were very motivational. Both of them advocate exercise, proper diet, and counseling to overcome whatever issues are holding people back from successfully sticking to a weight loss plan. Participants have to attend regular weigh-ins to keep track of their progress, helping them stay accountable to their goals. These contestants set their goals, developed their plan, made the commitment, stuck to it, and lost weight. **You can do the same!**

STEP 4: CHOOSE THE RIGHT NUTRITIONAL PLAN: LOW-CARB VERSUS LOW-FAT

Have you been on diets before, and then gained back the weight you lost? Do you wonder why your diet didn't work?

Fad diets simply don't work. You must have a long-term plan and stick to it, and the good news is that there are numerous reputable weight-loss programs that do work! In comparing them, their strategies often boil down to two main categories: low-carb diets and low-fat diets. A typical example of a good low-carb diet is the South Beach Diet. A typical example of a reputable low-fat diet is the Weight Watchers Diet. Based on pure theory, medical scientists recommend a low-fat diet for patients who have high lipid levels (cholesterol and triglycerides), and a low-carbohydrate diet for patients who do not. However, in practice, studies have shown that either type of diet will work for both groups of patients. Studies show that cholesterol and/or triglycerides decrease on either diet, too. **Actually, medical research shows that most reasonable and medically sound diets will yield good weight loss results if the patient will follow the diet, be consistent, and stay persistent.**

I recommend both plans to my patients, and recommend that each individual choose one that she likes, and feels that she can manage. Then, I recommend strong adherence and persistence with the chosen nutritional plan.

Many medical practitioners like the low carbohydrate option, and the South Beach Diet is a favorite. It is full of healthy foods, relatively easy to do, and it yields early, as well as long-term, measurable results. The South Beach Diet book suggests that the average person will lose 8 to 13 pounds in the first two weeks. While this may be a bit generous, most of my patients who aggressively follow the program do lose at least 4 to 6 pounds in the first two weeks. Much of this early weight loss comes from a change in metabolism and water loss. These early changes can translate into significant weight loss as the program progresses. I like the fact that my patients see a difference quickly with the South Beach Diet because an early success gives you confidence and enthusiasm about your weight loss, and helps you keep going towards your goal.

If you don't have time to prepare meals, consider the Nutrisystem® (nutrisystem.com) or JennyCraig® program (JennyCraig.com), **but—choose a diet and stay on it!**

In order to maintain long-term weight loss, you must have a permanent change in attitude about nutrition. If you don't, you will gain back all the weight that you lost, and probably even more. This is a well-known phenomenon. Don't let this happen to you. The concept of **mindfulness**, or awareness of what and how much you are eating, is very important to acquire. This is the time to re-train your mind in the concept of healthy nutrition.

Choose the South Beach Diet, or a low-carb diet of your choice, or the low-fat Weight Watchers Diet, and begin today!

STEP 5: MEASURE YOUR PORTION SIZES

It's not only what you eat, but how much. If you're going to eat healthily, lose weight, reshape your figure, and stay that way, you're going to have to come to terms with portion size. Whether you want to admit it or not, you know that portion size has gotten out of control in our society. The problem is, portion size itself has become so distorted that most of us don't even know what is normal anymore!

There are many ways to measure appropriate portions. The most accurate way would be to weigh all your food. This may be good in the beginning, but you will soon get tired of it. While I am very much in favor of weighing your food in the beginning so that you have an idea about accurate portion sizes, I recognize that most of you won't do it. The last thing you need is a reason for you not to be successful in this endeavor! So here is my easy rule of thumb for measuring portions:

For your entrée (the protein portion of your meal) make a fist with your hand. In general, that is a portion size!

Are You Too Hungry with Normal Portion Sizes?

I've had patients tell me that with normal portion sizes, they're still hungry. At first you might still feel hungry, as your body adjusts to a normal portion size. However, there are a few good habits you can implement to minimize that feeling of hunger.

- Most people don't chew their food well enough, and this leads to incomplete digestion, and a feeling of still being hungry. Make an effort to chew your food twice as long as you usually do.

- Drink more water. Most people don't drink nearly enough water, either, so make an effort to drink before and during your meal. Drink at least a glass of water with your meal, and consider a cup of herbal tea (without sugar!) after dinner. More fluids will give you a better feeling of fullness.

- It takes about 20 minutes after you've eaten for your body to have a feeling of fullness. Consequently, during a meal, we don't feel full until the very end of it, or even later.

Start using these good eating habits on yourself. Eat normal portion sizes, chew more, and drink more water. If you're still hungry, give yourself some time. You will be surprised that after 20 or 30 minutes, you won't feel hungry anymore.

STEP 6: CHOOSE YOUR EXERCISE PLAN

Perhaps you know you need to exercise, but you just can't get motivated to go to the gym, or to go out and walk every day. You are not alone, but you are going to need to change this if you are really going to make a change in your weight and your body shape. Increased physical activity must be part of your weight loss program. As with nutrition, many patients feel that they are exercising enough. Some of us are, but most of us aren't.

Exercise to Suit Your Needs

First, stay focused on your nutritional plan. Wait at least two weeks after you've implemented the changes in your diet before starting an exercise program. The reason for this is that it simply takes time for your body to adjust to your new nutritional program. As you are first adjusting, you're going to feel tired as your body undergoes a change in metabolism. You will adjust to this change after a couple of weeks and your energy will be restored.

Use these "two weeks off" to do some research on exercise programs that might fit your new lifestyle. I recommend that you pick up a few health magazines at the newsstand or pharmacy. There are some really good health magazines being published today, and they are loaded with great visual suggestions about good food, nutrition, and exercise programs. I like the magazines *Health, Natural Health, Prevention Magazine,* and *Mind, Body, & Spirit Fitness.* When you begin to read these magazines on a regular basis, you too will become health-conscious, and this adds to your enthusiasm about health, weight loss, and body reshaping.

Your two weeks are up and it's time to get moving! There are two types of exercise that are really necessary for you: weight-bearing or strength training, and aerobic. Where you begin with your exercise program depends on where you are now. If you are doing nothing, I recommend you start with walking every day. A great resource to track how long you are walking, or to pick a course, is www.mapmyrun.com. Using this website, you can input your start point and develop a walking course, turn by turn, and it will calculate the course's distance. As you feel your body getting into better shape, start to pick up the pace each day and add a few blocks to your walk. Keep a record of your daily exercise in your journal. At least 30 minutes of daily exercise is important, and it doesn't all have to be at one time. You can break it up over the course of the day, but remember that being persistent is necessary to success.

Don't forget to add things to your exercise program that you really like to do. For example, gardening, dancing, and even sex are excellent exercises.

The next step is to add some weight-bearing exercises. If you are not exercising at all, this can be a little harder. I recommend that you get some advice to begin with so that you won't hurt yourself. A good exercise program with some supervision is always best. If you have gone a long time without going to a gym, you might feel intimidated. It may be worthwhile to talk to a trainer at a gym and to discuss your fears. You might find that there are many people at the gym who have gone through a similar situation as you.

If you are really uncomfortable with a gym, there are great exercise DVD programs available at the bookstore. Here are two favorites of my patients:

- *Shrink Your Female Fat Zones* by Denise Austin
- *Prevention Personal Training* with Chris Freytag

Get one of these, and see if it appeals to you. Set aside 30 minutes every day for your DVD workout, and don't cheat! The benefit of the gym is that your trainer will be watching and you will be less likely to shirk off your workout! Don't shirk off at home either! I also recommend that you consider the book *Strong Women Stay Young* by Miriam Nelson, Ph.D. This is a very readable book. It is inexpensive, straight to the point, and will help you with your weight-bearing exercises.

Yoga and Pilates are also excellent body moving programs that can help exercise both body and mind. There are also highly respected DVD programs available at most bookstores. Consider one of these programs, also highly recommended by my patients.

- *Fat Burning Pilates* by Kathy Smith
- *Pilates Conditioning for Weight Loss* by Suzanne Deason
- *Pilates Target Specifics Plus* by Elizabeth Young
- *Power Yoga* by Kristin McGee

And don't forget to pick up those health magazines that will help keep you inspired and motivated! In addition to the general health magazines I've mentioned above, I'd recommend picking up a magazine that provides specific information about the exercise program you've decided upon. There are many magazines dedicated to yoga, Pilates, golf, tennis, swimming, running, and almost any other mode of exercise out there.

I strongly recommend at least 30 minutes of exercise every day. You can find the time, and it doesn't have to be done all at once.

STEP 7: TAKE ACTION!

This is the step that the majority of us fail to take! If you don't take action, you're going to stay the same weight (and probably gain) and will stay the same shape (or get larger). It doesn't have to be this way.

I know there is a good chance that you don't like the way you look and feel. While women come to my practice complaining of menopause symptoms every day (hot flashes, night sweats, etc.), **the number one complaint is weight gain and the inability to lose it**. In fact, this is the number one complaint of the majority of my patients, no matter what their menopausal status.

The simple fact is the physical law of thermodynamics has not changed. If you are to maintain your weight, the number of calories that you take in must equal the number of calories that you burn. If you gain weight over your lifetime this means that you have burned less than you have eaten. It is a simple physical law of the universe.

"The Perfect Menopause 7-step Weight Loss Plan" is the convergence of actions that I know are both successful and medically sound. It has worked with patients in my practice for over 25 years. **For each and every one of my patients for which this has worked, she has been committed and taken action.** If you don't put these concepts into action, it is unlikely that anything will change.

There is one last thing. If you have any significant medical problems, clear your diet plan and exercise plan with your menopause practitioner. No matter what your medical problem, it is unlikely that you will not be able to participate in some diet and exercise program. Let your menopause practitioner help guide you in that regard.

Remember Judy, the patient described at the beginning of this chapter? She had gained 40 pounds over eight years. Judy is a dietitian. She knew all the principles of healthy eating, calorie intake vs. burn, and the importance of a coach and support team. But she just never took action. Don't let this happen to you.

Take action and begin your program today! Do everything you can to maintain your program to reach your goals. And remember to journal your progress. If you put these principles into action, I guarantee that you will get a positive result.

E-mail me with your results. Your success will be my success too.

GET TO YOUR PERFECT WEIGHT

In Step 4 you've learned why weight can be easier to gain and harder to lose during menopause. You've also learned why it is so important to lose weight and keep it off during this time of your life. The benefits of weight loss go way beyond reducing hot flashes!

Step 4 also provided an action plan that you can use to lose weight healthily, and keep it off. Don't hesitate! You will probably live over a third of your life in menopause, and I'm willing to bet that you'd like be slim, trim, and healthy during these years! This is an important component to having "The Perfect Menopause."

In Step 5, you will be learning about aging and dryness. Your nutritional and exercise plan will help combat the effects of aging and dryness, so keep this in mind as you continue to read. Combating the effects and look of age is just one more fantastic reason to start your weight loss program today!

The Perfect Menopause Weight Loss Program

Baseline Data:

Name: _____   Waist: _____

Date: _____   Menopot: _____

Weight: _____   Breast: _____

Height: _____   Buttocks: _____

BMI: _____   Arm: _____

Blood Pressure: _____   Dress Size: _____

Lab Tests:

Cholesterol: Total: _____

Triglycerides: _____

HDL: _____

LDL: _____

Thyroid (TSH): _____

Fasting Glucose: _____

Blood Count (Hematocrit): _____

Weight and Body Shape Goals: Be Specific!

2 Weeks: _____

1 Month: _____

3 Months: _____

6 Months: _____

9 Months: _____

12 Months: _____

(Attach your picture!)

How Am I Going To Achieve This (Method)?

_____

_____

_____

_____

_____

_____

_____

_____

Progress Journal
Weight

Date/Week	Weight	Body Measurements	Progress Notes
1			
2			
3			
4			
5			
6			
7			
8			
9			
10			
11			
12			
13			
14			
15			
16			
17			
18			
19			
20			
21			
22			
23			
24			
25			
26			
27			
28			
29			
30			
31			

Progress Journal
Exercise

Date/Week	Exercise Progress	Documentation
1		
2		
3		
4		
5		
6		
7		
8		
9		
10		
11		
12		
13		
14		
15		
16		
17		
18		
19		
20		
21		
22		
23		
24		
25		
26		
27		
28		
29		
30		
31		

chapter

8

Step Five

Reverse Aging and Manage Your Dryness, Inside and Out

YOU MIGHT BE WONDERING what managing dryness has to do with aging. Dryness is one of the primary reasons women look older! Think about a grape versus a raisin . . . the grape, which is plump and juicy, looks young and fresh. The raisin, which is wrinkled and dry, just looks older. We humans are not that different from the grape. As we age, we dry out. As we dry out, we wrinkle and look older!

Consider Valerie's recent experience:

Valerie is a 49-year-old account executive at a major corporation. She had a hysterectomy and both ovaries removed at age 40 for endometriosis. She took estrogen for a year, and then stopped because of talk about cancer. Recently, during a job review with her boss, she was surprised to learn that he thought she was in her 60s.

For women who are in menopause, dryness leads to drastic changes of the skin, hair, and vagina. This is why it is important to manage dryness both inside and out. By doing so, you will also help to reverse (or at least slow down) wrinkling, hair loss, and vaginal atrophy.

SKIN

You might have looked in the mirror recently and thought, "I can't believe I look so old when I feel so young!" Imagine how you will look in five years, then 10 years. How has aging affected your mother's looks? How do you feel about this?

Changes in your estrogen level at perimenopause and menopause accelerate the physical changes in the skin that affect how you look and feel. No woman wants to look or feel old, so you want to take care of your skin for beauty and also for health.

Can you do anything to slow down the wrinkling process? Absolutely! Step 5 is about how you can reverse aging and dryness. Many menopause experts, as well as leading dermatologists, believe that dryness and skin aging is one of the most overlooked aspects of menopause and estrogen deprivation.

WHY IS SKIN DRYNESS, THINNING, AND WRINKLING, IMPORTANT TO YOU?

Your skin is your largest organ. It provides a covering for your major organs, and is a barrier to prevent injury and infection from entering other parts of your body. It is what shapes who you are physically. Like the body of your car, your skin is an essential component of your person, embodying your spirit and personality. Taking care of your skin is similar to keeping your front lawn beautiful. It takes a little time, but a lush, well-manicured lawn is often well worth the effort.

We know that drying, thinning, and wrinkling skin are natural consequences of aging and poor lifestyle choices, and that these aging effects are exacerbated by estrogen deprivation that begins at the perimenopause and menopause time. It takes only 1 to 3 years of lowered estrogen levels before significant effects to the skin are noted. After that, a woman's skin will age very rapidly, and changes to the skin will become very noticeable.

IS THE LACK OF ESTROGEN THE SECRET TO AGING SKIN?

We know that estrogen plays a major role in skin chemistry, physiology, and structure. Your skin is made up of three layers, the epidermis or outermost layer of skin, your dermis or middle layer of skin, and your subcutaneous (fat layer), the lowest layer of skin. The epidermis' primary functions are to provide skin pigmentation, to protect our inner organs, and to retain moisture. The dermis is where our hair follicles, nerves, blood vessels, sweat glands, and collagen and elastin reside. The subcutaneous layer or lowest layer is made up of loose connective tissue and fat (adipose) tissue.

The loss of estrogen at the menopause primarily causes a decrease in the production of collagen fibers and elastin in the dermis (middle layer), and the loss of these fibers decrease the volume of your skin. Decreased volume means thinner skin, and thinner skin leads to wrinkling. The decline in skin collagen with aging occurs at a greater rate during the first few years after menopause. Approximately 30% of skin collagen is lost in the first five years after menopause, and then the average collagen loss is 2.1% for each post menopause year after that. If you do the math, you will see that the average woman who begins her menopause at 51.4 years of age will have lost almost 40% of her skin's collagen by the time she is 60 years old. It is striking to know you will lose that much dimension to your skin so rapidly! (See Figure 8–1).

PHOTODAMAGE FROM THE SUN

Although the loss of hormones in the menopause plays a significant role in the aging of skin, there are other factors that cause damage as well. If you've ever seen a dermatologist, then I'm sure you've been warned about too much sun exposure. Photodamage from UV exposure (the sun) is very harmful to your skin. In addition to having a significant role in the development of skin cancer, UV exposure speeds up the process of skin degradation. UV radiation

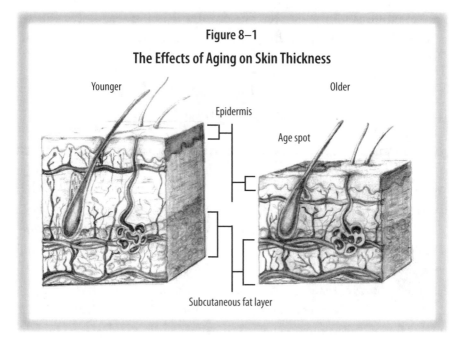

Figure 8–1

The Effects of Aging on Skin Thickness

Younger

Older

Epidermis

Age spot

Subcutaneous fat layer

causes the formation of free radicals, which leads to inflammation, damage to DNA, and damage to the cell membranes of the skin. This chain reaction ends with the breakdown of collagen.

There are ways to help prevent this, including the use of some natural substances. Retinoic acid, a naturally occurring derivative of vitamin A, is known to improve wrinkled skin. Evidence suggests it works by preventing many of the reactions in the skin that lead to photo-aging. Antioxidants are used to prevent photo-aging and the breakdown of collagen, elastin, and hyaluronic acid. Antioxidants have become very popular in the dermatology and skin care fields. Studies on rejuvenating antioxidants have supported the use of green tea, vitamin C, vitamin E, coenzyme Q_{10}, idebenone, lutein, lycopene, and even genistein, a phytoestrogen found in soy. These antioxidants can be applied topically or taken orally. Many skincare lines offer products that contain these ingredients.

OTHER LIFESTYLE FACTORS

For good skincare at menopause, lifestyle truly matters. If you smoke, stop immediately. Smoking is one of the most serious aggressors in the aging of skin. Smoking causes your blood vessels in your skin to get smaller, thereby making your skin drier. Smoking also releases free radicals directly into your blood stream, causing inflammation and damage to your skin and other organs. Remember, too, that smoking leads to a decrease in your body's natural estrogen production at much earlier ages. The effects of smoking on your skin are so pronounced, there is even a definition for "smoker's face." **If you smoke, you will age much sooner than normal in many ways, and it will be very obvious to you and others by the way your skin ages.**

Nutrition and hydration are very important factors in the maintenance of healthy, vigorous, and vital skin, and they should not be overlooked. You are what you eat, and if you eat poorly, your skin will manifest that. If you don't drink enough water, you will be dry and wrinkled like a raisin.

CAN ESTROGEN THERAPIES MAKE A POSITIVE DIFFERENCE IN MY SKIN?

Estrogen therapies, either in the form of skin creams or systemic therapies (oral or transdermal), can treat and/or prevent the damages that await your skin. If you are considering taking estrogen for your major menopausal symptoms, the aging of your skin may be an important benefit for you to factor into your decision.

Hormone skin creams have a long history in cosmetic dermatology. Like oral hormone therapies in the 1920s, hormone skin creams were the most popular "cosmeceutical" (cosmetic pharmaceutical) facial moisturizers. Both estrogen and progesterone creams were available in over-the-counter preparations. Then in 1930, the Cosmetics and Toiletries Act defined cosmetics as products that do not alter the structure or function of the skin. Hormone creams were then reclassified as drugs and a prescription became necessary to use a hormone cream. They are still used and prescribed by dermatologists today.

In the last 75 years, we have learned a lot about skin physiology and the effects of estrogen. We have abundant evidence that hormone therapy is effective for improving the appearance of aging skin. Estrogens improve skin rigidity, decrease wrinkling, and increase skin thickness as measured by many different parameters. When you lose estrogen, there is a decrease in your body's production of mucopolysaccharides and hyaluronic acid, both substances that are necessary for maintaining skin hydration. Decreased estrogen levels result in a decreased capillary blood flow in the skin. The resulting loss of collagen fibers, the dehydration of the skin, and decreased blood flow are all responsible for the thinning, drying, and wrinkling of your skin.

Many dermatologists claim they can immediately tell if a woman is taking hormone therapies there are significant difference in the skin's appearance before and after hormone therapy. The same dermatologists feel that hormone therapies are some of the best skin treatments available.

WILL A SIMPLE, VERY LOW-DOSE ESTROGEN CREAM HELP MY SKIN?

Yes, I believe it will. Many patients throughout the world use a very low-dose estrogen cream on the face, neck, and hands daily. There are some studies which show that even after 6 months, the elasticity and firmness of the skin are markedly improved, and wrinkle depth and pore sizes are decreased by 60–100%. Skin hydration is improved and collagen fibers are increased, as one could expect with the reintroduction of estrogen. The studies published thus far indicate that when doses are kept low, there is no increase in systemic estrogen levels from absorption, and no side effects.

THE PERFECT MENOPAUSE 7-STEP PLAN FOR THE PREVENTION AND TREATMENT OF DRY SKIN AT MENOPAUSE

While aging, sun exposure, our lifestyle choices, and estrogen deprivation are all working against your skin, there are many ways that you can keep skin wrinkling at a minimum, and even reduce the signs of wrinkling, without plastic surgery. The following 7-step plan will help you keep your skin vital during the menopause and postmenopause years:

Figure 8–2

The Perfect Menopause 7-Step Plan for the Prevention and Treatment of Dry Skin at Menopause

1. Correlate Your Skin Management With Your Other Therapies

2. Stay Hydrated

3. Use Supplements

4. Control Sun Exposure

5. Manage Lifestyle Factors

6. Use Hormones

7. Actively Manage All Your Medical Problems

---

1. Correlate your skin management with your other therapies. Involve your menopause practitioner. If you are already taking systemic estrogen, this may be enough. If you've opted for non-hormonal treatment or do not have other menopausal symptoms, your practitioner may refer you to a qualified dermatologist with an interest in the menopausal woman. A dermatologist may consider prescribing retinoic acid (Renova®, or Avage®). There are also prescription medications which contain collagen and hyaluronic acid. If your menopause practitioner feels it is warranted, such prescription medications for your skin may be very appropriate. The effort you put into this will pay great dividends down the road.

2. Stay hydrated. Most of us are in a constant state of dehydration. The older we get, the consequences of dehydration are more severe. And the more dehydrated you are, the more your skin will show it. Drink water and other appropriate fluids constantly. Keep in mind that some fluids such as alcoholic and caffeinated drinks are actually dehydrating. If you drink them, compensate by drinking more water throughout the day. Also remember that sodas, especially those containing carbonates and phosphates, draw calcium and magnesium from your bones! Even if you think you drink enough, you probably don't. In your menopause and post menopause years, the skin is thinner and fluids are lost through the skin more quickly.

Figure 8–3

Make Your Own Natural Oils Moisturizing Cream

Homemade Natural Oils Moisturizing Cream can be made using any of the essential oils of your choice. This recipe is adapted from Susan Belsinger, *The Herb Companion*, November 2006. There are many other similar formulas.

½ cup almond oil

½ cup grapeseed oil

½ cup cocoa butter

½ cup coarse grated natural beeswax, tight packed (about 1½ ounces)

1 teaspoon vitamin E oil

$1^{1}/_{3}$ cup distilled water

½ cup aloe vera gel

12–18 drops essential oil (your choice of essential oil or combinations. Lavender is a commonly used oil but others can be used alone or in combination)

Procedure:

In the top of a double boiler, combine the almond and grapeseed oils, cocoa butter and beeswax. Heat over medium heat until all has melted. Stir in vitamin E oil and let cool. When cooled to room temperature, transfer to a blender using a rubber scraper. It will be semisolid.

Combine distilled water and aloe in a measuring cup (room temperature) and add to the semisolid paste in the blender slowly, with the blender on low. The mixture will be very thick. Add the essential oils now as you blend. This will produce an emulsion. Blend for as long as is necessary at normal room temperature. Note: shake your emulsion before each use.

Keep the skin hydrated with moisturizing lotions. Apply lotion at least twice a day, in the morning and at night. Moisturizing lotions that contain antioxidants such as vitamin E, vitamin C, alpha lipoic acid, green tea, and coenzyme Q_{10}, are excellent for both moisturizing your skin and protecting it against further damage due to free radicals. Apply these lotions over your entire body.

Moisturizers using natural or essential oils are also available in health food stores, or you can make them yourself. See Figure 8–3 for formulas. These oils are not only natural, they are excellent moisturizing agents, and have an aroma that will truly invigorate your mind, body, and spirit.

During the winter, make sure you have a humidifier running. Dryness caused by heating systems in the wintertime can drain a considerable amount of water from your body, leaving your whole body very dry.

3. Use Supplements. There are a variety of supplements that are excellent antioxidants.

They can help in the prevention and treatment of photodamaged skin. Use the following supplements every day:

- A multivitamin
- Vitamin E—400 international units
- Fish oils—omega–3 fatty acids—1000 mg, two times per day.
- Coenzyme Q_{10}—30 mg
- B complex—50 mg
- Alpha lipoic acid—5200 mg

The multivitamin, Vitamin E, and Fish oils are also part of my recommended "The Perfect Menopause Natural Therapy Formula," so you may already be well on your way to improving your skin. If you are not using this formula, then begin these substances one at a time, and add one per week, every week. Remember, any vitamin has the potential to cause stomach upset, nausea or diarrhea. Beginning them one at a time will help isolate the problem should one occur.

4. Control sun exposure. The incidence of melanoma of the skin is rising rapidly among young sun worshipers. Even if you don't get melanoma, photodamage from ultraviolet rays can be a significant factor in early drying, wrinkling and thinning of the skin. **When the skin is already thinning, as in a postmenopausal woman, the effects of photodamage from the sun are more severe.**

Most people don't realize that when they cut the grass, work in the garden, or go to the market just a few blocks away, there is sun exposure. You are receiving ultraviolet (UV) radiation doing your daily chores, just as you would on the beach. Using a tanning bed is even worse for your skin because the ultraviolet radiation penetrates into the dermis layer of the skin, causing deeper damage.

The best thing you can do to protect your skin is to limit sun exposure. Wear a hat and sunscreen every time you go outside. Use a 30 SPF broad-spectrum sunscreen which protects the skin from UVA and UVB rays. Reapply your sunscreen every 90 minutes to be cautious. The cosmetics industry has introduced many new facial moisturizers that contain sunscreen agents. If you are using one of these products, be careful to choose one that protects you from a broad spectrum of UV radiation. Talk to your dermatologist for a product or brand recommendation.

5. Manage lifestyle factors. Lifestyle factors play an extremely important role in the management of your skin.

- **Smoking**: The most important lifestyle factor to change is smoking. Smoking can have devastating effects on all aspects of your body, and your skin is no exception. Smoking can lead to an earlier onset of menopause, lower levels of estrogen and decreased blood flow to the skin. This all contributes to dry, thin, and wrinkled skin at an earlier age. You will look older more quickly if you smoke.

- **Exercise, Sleep, and Nutrition**: Exercise is necessary for every aspect of your health. Exercise increases blood flow to all organs of your body, bathing all of your organs in increased levels of oxygen and nutrients which are essential for your skin health. Studies have shown that proper rest and sleep are also necessary for the maintenance of a healthy skin. When you sleep, you give your cells the chance to regenerate. Also, it should be obvious that proper nutrition is important in maintaining good skin. Nutrients necessary for healthy skin will not be obtained without proper nutrition. This is another reason to consider the advice given in Chapter 7. You wouldn't deny your lawn of the proper fertilizer and water, so keep your skin properly moisturized and nourished also!

6. Use Hormones. Do you take estrogen now? Are you wondering if you should keep taking it? For aging skin, low-dose estrogen benefits you!

Estrogen therapies are the most successful of all therapies for the management of skin aging. Many women dismiss estrogen skin creams just because they are "opposed to estrogen." I hope you will read everything in this book about the most current and up-to-date thinking about estrogen before you completely rule out topical estrogen treatments. Getting all the correct knowledge may make all the difference in your decision.

If you are currently taking hormones and are thinking about going off of them, you owe it to yourself to consider the impact to your skin in your decision. Certainly, you will want to develop a skin-treatment plan to address the changes that going off of hormones will instigate. If you are not taking estrogen, **consider the use of a very low-dose estrogen skin cream to treat your skin without systemic absorption**. If you choose this method, I recommend hormone testing before therapy, and then again after 3 months of treatment. The purpose of the testing is to be sure that there has been no absorption of the estrogen contained in the cream into your blood stream.

Estrogen Cream for Skin Therapy

Estrogen cream for the skin is not available commercially. However, it can be obtained with a prescription through a compounding pharmacy. Use a cream with 0.3% estriol in aqua glycolic acid (3 mg of estriol/g aqua glycolic acid), or 0.01% estradiol, also in aqua glycolic acid. Research shows that these strengths are effective and safe. Apply small amounts daily to your face, neck, and hands. NOTE: Many gynecologists aren't familiar with these creams or doses, but may be willing to prescribe them based on my recommendations in this book. Share this with her/him.

7. Actively manage all your medical problems. Active management of any other medical problems you may have is very important in the management of your skin. If you have diabetes, hypertension, or other medical problems, keeping them in control with appropriate management will have a direct influence on the healthfulness and vitality of your skin in the menopause and postmenopause time. Some medical problems can be complex. Be sure to discuss how your other medical issues may impact your skin's health with your menopause practitioner.

Follow these seven important steps, and I guarantee that
your skin will look and feel more vital and youthful!

HAIR LOSS, DRYNESS, AND BRITTLENESS

Are you finding larger and larger amounts of hair in your shower drain? And have you noticed that your hair is drier and more brittle? Hair is an integral part of your skin, and many of the same concepts described above about aging, menopause, and the effects of estrogen deficit to your skin also apply to your hair.

There is a normal amount of hair loss that can be expected for all women. A clump of hair in your shower drain about the size of a quarter (depending on how long you wear your hair, of course) every week is normal for a woman at any age. This hair loss is all part the natural lifecycle of the hair and it will regenerate. In the late perimenopause and menopause ages, hair loss is accelerated, and you can expect to find larger clumps of hair in the drain. The amount of hair loss will vary depending on your genetics, and how you manage your menopause. Taking special care of your hair and using high-quality products to wash and condition your scalp and hair will minimize hair loss, and keep your hair and scalp feeling and looking healthy. Figure 8–4 outlines some basic tips to follow in order to maintain beautiful and healthy hair.

If you feel you have excessive hair loss, it is important that you work with your menopause provider to evaluate this problem. There are three primary types of hair loss in females: telogen effluvium, alopecia areata, and female androgenic alopecia. Therapeutic recommendations are different depending on the type of hair loss. Understanding of the types of hair loss will help you discuss this with your menopause provider.

1. Telogen effluvium. This type of hair loss is characterized by diffuse thinning where a greater than normal number of hair follicles enter the resting phase, or "telogen phase," of hair loss. It is often caused by stress or hormonal changes, and the hair loss is usually noticed only a few months after the causative event. This type of hair loss usually resolves on its own within six months.

Telogen effluvium can be caused by hormonal changes such as thyroid disorders, or sudden hormonal changes such as a hysterectomy, or cessation of estrogen therapy. Other causes include surgery, major trauma, chronic

---

Figure 8–4

Hints On How To Manage Your Dry Scalp and Hair During Menopause

- Consult your personal hair stylist about your individual hair and scalp needs.
- Know that most menopausal women have dry scalp to such an extent that it is called "dead scalp."
- Most gray hair (and gray hair is the norm at menopause) is dry and porous, and it needs special moisturizing attention.

The world's hair experts recommend the following for the menopause woman:

- Massage your scalp frequently. It feels good and loosens up the dead scalp.
- Brush your hair frequently. This also loosens up the dead scalp and helps natural oils move through the hair.
- Always shampoo twice—once to get off dead skin and get rid of hair products; the second to thoroughly cleanse your scalp and hair.
- For very dry, "dead scalp," use Tea Tree Oil Shampoo.
- For a heavy buildup from hair products, or after swimming in a pool, use a clarifying shampoo.
- Use a light conditioner, especially with gray, porous hair. Heavy conditioners can weigh your hair down. Never put a conditioner directly on the scalp.
- The sun and heat (including blow drying) makes hair, especially gray hair, drier. Use light, spray products specifically designed to protect hair from damage due to the sun and heat.

---

illnesses, high fever, anorexia, and medicines such as beta blockers, antico-agulants, retinoids, and gout medications. This type of hair loss also is found in people who are nutritionally deficient, especially those with deficiencies in iron, zinc, and protein.

Correction of hormonal and nutritional imbalances, and patience, are often the best therapies.

2. Alopecia areata. This is another common type of hair loss—it manifests by sudden, patchy, hair loss. Alopecia areata is thought to be caused by a defect in the immune system which causes it to attack the hair follicles. This type of hair loss is sometimes associated with women who have autoimmune diseases, such as lupus, but it is often seen by itself, too. When alopecia areata is diagnosed, it can be treated with steroids, and the bald patches usually fill back in. The bald patches often fill in by themselves without the steroids, but this takes longer.

3. Female androgenic alopecia. Also called "female baldness pattern," this is the most common type of hair loss, and it is the most frustrating to treat. It is a gradual, diffuse, overall thinning of the hair at the crown of the head. Thought to be genetically inherited, it affects more than 10% of perimeno-pausal women, and up to 75% of those over age 65. It is caused by the presence of the hormone dihydrotestosterone, which is the same androgenic hormone that causes male pattern baldness. Female androgenic alopecia affects the size of the hair follicle and growth phases of the hair. In women, hormonal changes frequently exacerbate proper hair follicle growth, and some women even notice symptoms when using oral contraceptives.

The only FDA-approved treatment for female androgenic alopecia is Rogaine® (2% topical minoxidil). It takes three to six months of treatment before it begins to work, but hair usually does grow back to some extent. It is estimated that Rogaine stimulates moderate re-growth of hair in 19% of women and minimal re-growth in another 40% of women. Unfortunately, Rogaine doesn't help in either of the other types of hair loss.

Other Options

For female androgenic alopecia, some physicians prescribe anti-androgen drugs such as Propecia® and Proscar®. However, both of these drugs have considerable side effects, including breast tenderness, breast enlargement, nausea and a significant decrease in libido. When the hair loss is consider-able and thyroid levels are normal, other treatment options include a trial of hormone therapy (preferably bioidentical estrogen/progesterone) to oppose and block the dihydrotestosterone, and a high-potency daily multivitamin and mineral supplement.

Dr. Julian Whitaker is a well-known and respected medical doctor who runs a wellness clinic in California. Dr. Whitaker is an advocate of integrated medicine (combining allopathic or regular medicine with alternative/natural methods). He reports in his "Health and Healing" newsletter that a device called The Hairmax LaserComb™ has shown promise for all types of hair losses. This comb harnesses the energy of certain wavelengths of light to stim-ulate increased blood flow to the hair follicles. You simply comb through your hair three times a week for 10 minutes each time. Many women report having thicker, fuller hair in 8 to 16 weeks. The cost of the comb is $545, but if you aren't satisfied, there is 100% money back guarantee if you return it within 90 days. You can find out more about it at www.lasercomb.net. I respect Dr. Whitaker's knowledge and insight. Several of our patients have tried the laser-comb and have found it useful. But if you try it and it doesn't work after 90 days, return it and get your refund.

VAGINAL DRYNESS, THINNING WALLS, AND PAINFUL INTERCOURSE

Significant vaginal atrophy (thinness and dryness of the vaginal walls) and painful intercourse almost always occur as a result of estrogen deficiency in menopause. While hot flashes, night sweats, and mood dysfunction frequently improve, and even bone loss slows down as time progresses past the menopause, vaginal atrophy usually gets worse with time.

Consider the situations of these three women. Do any of their issues sound familiar to you?

Susan:

Susan is a 54-year-old woman who recently told me she feels totally dried up like a prune. She told me that she "doesn't feel female anymore" and that she "feels half dead inside." Intimacy with her husband is almost impossible due to her condition, and she feels sorry for him. She has tried vaginal moisturizers for the dryness, and they have helped somewhat. Susan and her husband have tried various lubrication products for intimacy. This makes it more slippery, but there is still intense pain during intercourse. She asked me if there was anything else she could do to help regain moisture and be able to enjoy her sex life again.

Susan's symptoms are all too common among menopausal women. Symptoms of vaginal atrophy can include feelings of vaginal dryness, pressure, genital burning and itching, urinary urgency, and sometimes frequent bladder and vaginal infections. Painful intercourse almost always results.

Structurally, vaginal atrophy is very similar to the thinning and wrinkling of the skin. It results from the breakdown of collagen, smooth muscle, and elastin, all of which are building blocks of the tissues of the vagina and pelvis. The tissue right at the opening of the vagina (known as the introitus) contains a high amount of collagen, smooth muscle and elastin. **With atrophy, this tissue becomes so thin it no longer is able to stretch and expand**, making intercourse impossible. Without intervention, the vaginal opening becomes very narrow and small, and very difficult to open. This is known as introital stenosis.

Mary:

Mary is a 49-year-old single woman who never married, and was never sexually active. There is a very high incidence of breast, ovarian, and uterine cancer in her family. As a result, Mary had a hysterectomy at age 40, and both of her ovaries were removed. She never took estrogen.

Recently, Mary has fallen in love and plans on getting married. But she has discovered that sexual intercourse is impossible. Examination shows that she has severe introital stenosis from nine years of estrogen deprivation as well as the lack of sexual activity. Because of this marked vaginal atrophy and stenosis, it took nine months of treatment with an estrogen vaginal cream, as well as the daily use of vaginal dilators, before Mary was able to be intimate with her new husband.

Jane:

Jane is a 54-year-old woman who has not had intercourse since her divorce over five years ago. She has never used hormones. Recently, she has been dating a gentleman who uses Viagra. In their first intercourse, she suffered tremendous pain and bleeding from tearing.

In addition to the breakdown of collagen, smooth muscle, and elastin, there is also a decrease in blood flow to the vagina and other pelvic organs with atrophy, which leads to increased difficulty in achieving sexual arousal and orgasms. Women with thin, dry tissues that contain fewer blood vessels in the vaginal walls have an increased risk of physical injury during sexual activity. In addition to the painful intercourse, bleeding may occur. Not only can this be painful, but it can increase your sensitivity to acquiring a sexually transmitted disease. As more women are becoming single and beginning to date during the perimenopause and menopause years, vaginal atrophy and its long-term effects can be a significant concern.

Estrogen deprivation is the leading cause of vaginal dryness and subsequent atrophy during the perimenopause and menopause years. But there can be other factors that may exacerbate this or accentuate it sooner. Certain medications, such as antihistamines and some (tricyclic) antidepressants, can cause vaginal drying to be more pronounced and even lead to atrophy earlier. Women with Sjogren's syndrome have significant vaginal dryness as well as dryness of the eyes and mouth, and may experience even more dryness than other women at the perimenopause and menopause.

Birth control pills can also cause some vaginal dryness, and some younger women are also bothered by this. Birth control pills contain synthetic estrogens and progestins and work by reducing natural estrogens in your body. Some of the very low-dose birth control pills can cause enough reduction in your natural estrogens to cause a symptomatic vaginal dryness.

WHAT CAN YOU DO TO TREAT THE SYMPTOMS OF VAGINAL DRYNESS, THINNESS, AND ATROPHY?

Many of the strategies used to treat dry skin also apply to treating vaginal dryness. Maintaining a healthy lifestyle, keeping hydrated, and taking vitamins and supplements will help. Maintaining a regular and satisfying intimate life will also help keep the vaginal walls vascularized and vital.

There are many products that are marketed as vaginal moisturizers to help with generalized comfort, and many lubricants to help with intimacy. (See Figure 8–5.) These products may be helpful, but you should be careful what you insert into your vagina at this time. Substances that stick to the vaginal walls increase the likelihood of infections. Most over-the-counter vaginal moisturizers are water-based and do not adhere to the vaginal walls, which is preferable. Moisturizers such as Gyne-Moistrin®, Replens®, or Vitamin E oil, are ideal vaginal moisturizers. I recommend that patients use a vaginal moisturizer regularly, at least every other day, to keep the vaginal walls as vital as possible. Expected results with the regular use of vaginal moisturizers are similar to that of skin moisturizers. They should help with generalized comfort as well as maintain the vitality of the vaginal tissues.

Figure 8–5
Water Soluble Vaginal Moisturizers and Lubricants

Product	Moisturizer	Lubricant
Replens®	✓	
Gyne-Moistrin®	✓	
Coconut oil	✓	✓
Vitamin E oil	✓	✓
AstroGlide®		✓
K-Y® Jelly Lubricant		✓
Sensua® Organics Personal Lubricant		✓
Sacred Moments® Intimate Infusions		✓
O'My® Natural Lubricants		✓
Arkadia™ [1]	✓	✓

[1] www.myarkadia.com

Moisturizers containing natural oils can be great for vaginal dryness, and have recently become commercially available (Arkadia line of moisturizers and lubricants). You can also easily make one. I recommend the formula in Figure 8–6. Natural oils are a little bit pricey, but the results will be worth it. They are soothing, revitalizing, and the aroma produced will invigorate your mind, body, and spirit.

There are also many vaginal lubricants available for use during intimacy. It is important to realize that vaginal lubricants are different than moisturizers.

Figure 8–6

Essential Oil Vaginal Rejuvenation Cream You Can Make Yourself

- 2 ounces almond oil or vegetable oil
- 6 drops each of rose geranium and lavender essential oils
- 1500 international units of vitamin E oil (liquid or open a capsule)
- 1 drop of neroli essential oil (expensive, so it is optional)

Combine ingredients. For the vitamin E, use either the liquid vitamin or pop open a couple of capsules and empty out the contents. Apply as needed inside the vagina.

Vaseline®, coconut oil, vitamin E oil, Astroglide®, Today®, and Arkadia are all great lubricants. Check the ingredients of other lubrication products carefully. Petroleum-based products and products that contain animal or synthetic glycerin can cause irritation and yeast infections. Petroleum-based products cannot be used with latex condoms because they weaken the latex, so be careful when choosing your lubricant if you also plan to use a condom.

The act of intimacy itself is an important way to keep your vaginal walls vascularized, vital and well moisturized. This is one area where the old adage "use it or lose it" definitely holds true! Sexual intercourse promotes blood flow to the vaginal walls, which helps keep your vaginal walls vascularized, moisturized, and bathed in nutrients. You may need to be careful at first if it has been a while since you have been intimate. But it is a good idea to keep up as normal a sex life as possible in order to maintain vaginal vitality.

Don't rule out the use of a very small amount of
vaginal estrogen cream or other local therapies.

There probably is no other area of your body where the role of estrogen is so important as it is to the vagina. Like skin dryness, the manifestations of the vaginal dryness and subsequent atrophy often take a few years to be significant. When they do become significant, vaginal moisturizers and lubricants alone frequently don't provide enough relief if a woman is expecting to continue to have a satisfactory intimate life. If intimacy is not an issue, then vaginal atrophy may not be a problem unless dryness is causing vaginal discomfort or other symptoms like frequent bladder and vaginal infections.

The most effective way to treat severe vaginal atrophy is via localized estrogen therapy. The good news is that local therapy, which is a very small amount of low-dose estrogens applied directly to the vagina, can usually treat and/or reverse vaginal atrophy significantly enough that vaginal discomfort is virtually non-existent and a reasonable, even pleasurable, intimate life is possible.

When many women were still taking systemic estrogen therapy, before the results from WHI 2002 were reported, most women were prescribed oral estrogens at much higher doses than we are accustomed to using today. As a result, there was a lower incidence of vaginal atrophy than there is today. Now, women either prefer not to use systemic estrogen therapy, or are using significantly lower doses of systemic estrogen to manage their menopausal symptoms. Consequently, these doses often aren't enough to ensure vaginal health for sexually active women, and local vaginal therapies may be necessary. There are 3 types of very low-dose local estrogen therapy available:

1. Vaginal creams
2. Vaginal tablet
3. Vaginal ring

See Figure 8–7 for details about brand names and active ingredients for each of these types of local therapies.

Figure 8–7
Vaginal Estrogen Therapies

Product	Estrogen Component
Vagifem® Vaginal Tablets	Estradiol[1]
Estring® Vaginal Ring	Estradiol[1]
Estrace® Vaginal Cream	Estradiol[1]
Premarin® Vaginal Cream	Conjugated Estrogens[2]
Bijuva™ Vaginal Cream	Conjugated Estrogens[1]
Estriol Vaginal Cream	Estriol[3]

1. Plant derived
2. Pregnant mare urine derived
3. Compound pharmacies in USA

Each product has a different treatment protocol, and therapy should be individualized to your personal situation. The vaginal tablet (Vagifem®) contains a mere 25 micrograms of estradiol, the bioidentical estrogen produced by the ovary. It comes with a vaginal applicator and is dispensed by the patient deep into the vagina where it dissolves, working directly on the vaginal tissues. For the average patient, recommended dosing is one pill daily for approximately 2 weeks, then one pill every other day thereafter.

The vaginal ring (Estring®) also contains a low dose of estradiol. It is easily placed into the vagina by the patient, and the estrogen is slowly released into the vagina over a three-month period. Most patients do not feel the ring, even during intercourse.

The vaginal estrogen creams are often preferred by the patient, and are the most commonly used. There are two prescription brands available, and another that will soon be available. Premarin® vaginal cream and Estrace® cream are both currently available by prescription. Premarin vaginal cream's active ingredients are the conjugated equine estrogens found in the oral pill. Estrace contains the bioidentical estradiol. Both come with a vaginal applicator, and a common dose is 1 gram of cream at bedtime, two to three times per week. Bijuva® is a new estrogen cream in the late stage of clinical trials. Plant derived, Bijuva has a mixture of estrogens and may be able to be used effectively in even smaller amounts than other available creams.

Various other estrogen vaginal creams are also available through compounding pharmacies. One particular favorite is estriol vaginal cream. Estriol is a bioidentical in that it is produced by the human body, but only in the smallest amounts (except in pregnancy when it is produced in much larger amounts). Compared to estradiol, it is a very weak estrogen (see Chapter 3). But for local vaginal therapy, it works well for many patients. The dose is 0.5 mg of estriol per gram of cream, and it is used as one gram of cream 2–3 times per week, after an initial use of every night for two weeks.

All of the vaginal products contain very low doses of estrogen, and are meant for local (vaginal) therapy only. They are not strong enough to provide help for other menopause related issues such as hot flashes and night sweats. Studies are limited, but the data show that with local estrogen therapies a small amount of estrogen may be absorbed by the very thin vaginal walls. In this circumstance, a woman might notice some slight breast tenderness initially. However, as the vaginal walls begin to thicken, the likelihood of significant systemic absorption is reduced. Although controversial, some menopause experts believe that because there is minimal absorption, very low dose estrogen vaginal therapies may be considered in some patients with breast cancer who have finished their breast cancer therapies.

MY RECOMMENDATIONS

Although I recommend all of the vaginal estrogen therapies depending on the circumstances, I often prefer the estrogen vaginal cream because it does not need to be placed deep into the vaginal canal. Vaginal creams also allow my patients some flexibility in their dosing that other therapies can't provide. I often advise my patients to forget using the applicator and to apply a toothpaste-sized dose (about ¼ teaspoon) of the cream to their vagina using the end of their finger. This way, the end of the finger can be placed just inside the vaginal opening (introitus) just at the spot where the cream is needed, and briefly massaged in while gently stretching the vaginal tissues.

This application method provides both a small amount of estrogen and a bit of manual therapy to the most significantly affected tissue. (See Figure 8–8.) Brief stretching induces growth and elasticity. We recommend patients do this at least every other night, and sometimes every night, depending on the circumstances. When applied at bedtime, the small amount of estrogen will also roll back into the deeper portions of the vagina through the night. This technique, when used frequently and consistently, helps tremendously to reverse vaginal atrophy and maintain good vaginal health. A useful hint: when there are longer intervals of sexual abstinence, keep the vaginal walls healthy by continuing to use the vaginal estrogen and the blood flow active by frequent vaginal massage with your fingers or a vibrator. This practice will pay long term dividends. The company Arkadia™ has a very reputable safe, and useful line of intimate enhancement products (www.myarkadia.com).

REVERSE AGING AND DRYNESS, INSIDE AND OUT

In Step 5 we've learned that menopause and aging rapidly affects the dryness of our skin, hair, and vaginal tissues. Estrogen receptors are located in

Figure 8–8

Fingertip Application Method for Estrogen Cream

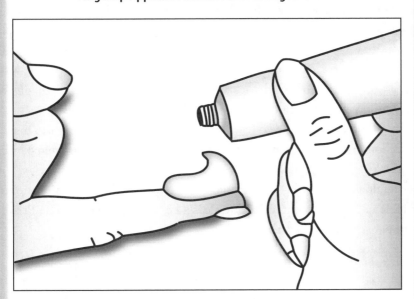

1. Wash your hands with soap and water and dry thoroughly.
2. Squeeze out a toothpaste size amount (about enough to cover the tip of your index finger, from the last joint to the finger tip).
3. Place estrogen cream and finger just inside the vagina and gently massage.
4. Apply at bed time.

Caution: Estrogen vaginal cream should not be used as a vaginal lubricant for intimacy. It is not slippery enough, and when this cream is used just prior to intimacy, there may be some transference to your partner. When intimacy is anticipated, skip the estrogen cream that night or apply it later.

Occasional intimacy directly after application of the cream is okay. Spontaneity itself should be respected as highly healing in many ways. For routine use, do not use vaginal estrogen cream just prior to intercourse.

every organ of the body, and the reduction in estrogen will affect all organs. This means that your skin and vaginal tissue will only reflect the state of health of your total body. Inner dryness can lead to more rapid aging and body dysfunction, consequences of aging that may be significantly reduced by paying closer attention to this state of dryness. Increased dryness of the mouth, eyes and nose, changes in bowel movements and gastrointestinal function, all are manifestations of this dryness. Our hands and feet begin to dry and crack, our nails become more brittle, our scalps more flaky, and our hair thinner and dryer.

It is obvious that if this dryness is occurring throughout your body, even more vital organs will be affected. Can your brain, heart, and lungs operate at peak efficiency and live long lives as they become more and more dehydrated?

Let the information that you learned in this chapter make you more aware of all aspects of your body's dryness. Use all the information in this chapter to help you stay vital, healthy, and hydrated. **Be a grape, not a raisin!**

In Step 6, we're going to learn more about sexuality during the menopause. You've learned about how to deal with vaginal atrophy in Step 5. Step 6 will address that and other issues related to sexuality, such as revving up your libido and achieving orgasms. For many women, the ability to continue having a satisfying and fulfilling sex life is a key factor in having **The Perfect Menopause**.

chapter

9

Step Six
Dramatically Improve Your Sexual Desire

Do Mara's comments sound familiar to you?

Mara is 47 years old, married, and has two teenaged children. She has begun to have mildly irregular periods and some night sweats, but her most significant complaint is her complete lack of sexual desire. "I love my husband. I don't want it to be like this."

Next to weight gain, the second most common complaint of my patients is their loss of sexual desire. A lack of sexual fulfillment is a common and frustrating problem for many women at menopause, and it can be related to many issues, both physical and emotional. When it comes to sex, the lack of desire is the most common complaint, followed by painful intercourse due to dryness. Difficulty with orgasms is the third most frequent complaint. Maybe you've experienced one or more of these issues yourself.

What is behind your lack of sexual desire and fulfillment? There are seven major factors that could potentially be involved in the cause(s):

1. Decreased hormone levels
2. Decreased blood flow due to age
3. Other medications
4. General health issues
5. A stale emotional relationship
6. A stale intimate relationship
7. Loss of communication

You might be surprised by some of the causes on this list. They may be things you hadn't thought about, or maybe didn't want to think about. Whether the reasons for your lack of sexual desire are due to hormonal changes at menopause, or due to a relationship that isn't quite what it should be, there are ways to go about remedying each of these issues and reclaiming your sexuality.

1. Decreased Hormone Levels

Are hormones behind your lack of sexual desire and fulfillment? Most women who discuss a lack of sexual fulfillment with me feel that it is due to hormonal changes related to menopause. This is a legitimate concern as the estrogen and testosterone ratios change dramatically at menopause for women (but change much, much less in men).

Estrogen levels in women typically decrease throughout the perimenopause and become very low after menopause. Testosterone also decreases over time. Only a few men and women abruptly lose significant levels of testosterone, and fall below the lowest normal level. For these men and women, this is a situation known as **andropause** (For more information, refer to Chapter 2).

We know that testosterone is the hormone of desire. Both men and women have testosterone, and while women have much lower levels of testosterone and much larger levels of estrogen than men, both sexes have and need both hormones. Testosterone levels in women are important not only for sexual function, but for overall well-being too. A woman whose testosterone level is too low will not only have decreased sexual desire, but may also not feel well in general. She may experience increased levels of fatigue, depression, or notice a decreased ability to concentrate and focus.

Some women at the perimenopause and/or menopause time have lowered levels of testosterone. Other women experience decreased receptor sensitivity, which means that their normal levels may not affect receptor sites as effectively as they used to. Either issue can noticeably affect a woman's libido and/or sexual function.

What are your normal testosterone levels? This is a key question to ask, yet a difficult one to answer. The normal range of testosterone levels is quite broad, which is one of the reasons why an excess or deficiency is difficult to measure. The average adult woman has somewhere between 50 to 70 ng (nanograms) of testosterone/dL (deciliter) of blood plasma. For comparison, the average adult male has a testosterone level of somewhere between 260 and 1,000 ng/dL. Each person's body chemistry is so unique, that a woman whose testosterone level is at the low end of the range may have enough for her function, but the next woman whose testosterone level is at the high end of normal may still have a deficiency with respect to her body's needs.

Testosterone does not act alone in either men or women. Estrogen is also necessary. The ancient Chinese concept of Yin-Yang, where two seemingly opposite things compliment each other to make a whole depicts the delicate hormone balance that affects a woman's physical and emotional well-being and sexual health. Here is a summary of what we know about the chemistry and biology of love:

1. Sexual interest or libido is related to enough testosterone reaching brain receptors. Low levels of testosterone may result in the cognitive sensation of decreased sexual interest or desire.

2. Sexual pleasure and sensitivity is heightened for both men and women when testosterone levels are at their peak.

3. Sexual orgasm is enhanced for both men and women by testosterone.

4. Attraction and arousal are linked with male and female body odors or pheromones. A person who is low in testosterone will produce fewer pheromones, resulting in less attraction and arousal of their mate.

5. For women, sexual receptivity and desire are at their peak when estrogen levels peak during the menstrual cycle. They are at their lowest during menses, when estrogen levels are at their lowest levels.

6. Both estrogen and testosterone are important for a woman to maintain lubrication, sensitivity, and integrity of the vagina, labia, and clitoris.

7. Romance alters a woman's biochemistry. A woman's testosterone level rises during the first few months of a relationship, while a man's falls off. These changes are usually temporary, and testosterone levels usually return to a more normal level after 1–2 years of the relationship.

8. Sexual fulfillment is also related to oxytocin, a hormone produced by the pituitary gland. Oxytocin levels rise dramatically during orgasm, enhancing sensitivity of the skin and sexual organs. Oxytocin also increases the feeling of sexual bonding. It is known as the "feel good" hormone. The effects of oxytocin are enhanced by estrogen, but dampened by too much testosterone.

9. Testosterone levels slowly decline in both men and women as we age. While estrogen levels dramatically decline in menopause, testosterone levels typically do not.

HUMAN SEXUALITY IS VERY COMPLEX

The human sexual response is very complex and sensitive to many factors. Hormonally, there is a very delicate balance that needs to be maintained between estrogen and testosterone levels for optimum sexual response in both men and women. But most women have significantly reduced estrogen levels at menopause, and it is the loss of estrogen that frequently is the cause of the sexual dysfunction. **For most women in this situation, supplementation with estrogen leads to a significant improvement in desire and sexual function.**

MODE OF ESTROGEN DELIVERY CAN BE IMPORTANT

Oral estrogens have a unique property in that they can increase the amount of a protein in the blood called sex hormone binding globulin (SHBG). SHBG binds with free testosterone, which can decrease the amount of free testosterone available in the blood for action. It is the free, or unbound, testosterone which is effective in the blood. Consequently, when libido or sexual dysfunction issues are significant, transdermal or transvaginal estrogens are the preferred therapies. Transdermal and transvaginal estrogens bypass the liver in their first pass through the body, and therefore don't significantly increase the production of sex hormone binding globulin (SHBG). This means that there is more free testosterone available for action when a transdermal or transvaginal estrogen is used.

WHEN IS TESTOSTERONE SUPPLEMENTATION APPROPRIATE?

In certain women, testosterone supplementation for decreased sexual desire/decreased sexual function is an appropriate option for therapy. In my practice, I request blood tests first to determine current serum levels of estradiol, estrone, and free testosterone. It is important to know the level of free testosterone, rather than the total testosterone, because it is the free testosterone that is the active hormone. A normal total testosterone level isn't meaningful if the free testosterone level is too low. When getting your hormone levels tested, it is important to go to a laboratory known to measure free testosterone levels accurately. Not all laboratories can do this. Your experienced menopause provider will recommend the best place to go in your community.

Recall that most women will have a testosterone level in the normal range, even if they experience decreased sexual desire. But at menopause, the estrogen levels are usually low, which is often the cause of the hormonal imbalance. For therapy, I first recommend considering a low dose of a transdermal bioidentical estradiol product. If, after 3 months of therapy, the desire is not improved, I would then consider testosterone supplementation.

Why would the testosterone supplementation work when the testosterone levels are in the normal range? This question has been asked for many years. And for a long time, we tended not to treat women with testosterone who had normal testosterone levels. However, recent clinical evidence has shown that some women in this situation do respond to testosterone supplementation. Either their testosterone levels are much lower at menopause than they were when they were younger, or their receptor sites require higher levels to be activated appropriately.

IF YOU NEED TO TAKE TESTOSTERONE, HERE'S HOW TO DO IT

I prefer to use bioidentical testosterone. Unfortunately, there is not a current pharmaceutical testosterone preparation available for women. A transdermal testosterone patch is under investigation, and hopefully will be available in the near future. Until then, bioidentical testosterone preparations must be obtained from a reliable compounding pharmacy. My recommendation is to use a transdermal cream or gel on the arm, vulvar lips, or preferably to the vagina. When used vaginally, the testosterone further improves blood flow to the vaginal and vulvar tissues, aiding in sexual response. This is described in Figure 9–1.

If you prefer an oral preparation, micronized bioidentical testosterone is also available from compounding pharmacies. Oral testosterone is rapidly absorbed, and therefore needs to be taken twice daily in order to maintain a continuous, therapeutically active blood level. Directions on how I recommend using oral testosterone are also detailed in Figure 9–1.

There are potential side effects that can result from having too much testosterone. Most women do not experience side effects. But if you do experience side effects, they usually are due to too much testosterone. If side effects are noted, they can include facial acne, (usually the first sign of too much testosterone) increased skin oiliness, and mild facial hair growth. With significantly higher levels of testosterone, increased facial hair, loss of scalp hair, and a deepening voice can be noted. These more serious side effects are very unusual.

Figure 9–1

Directions for Testosterone Supplementation for Women

All Testosterone Supplements Below are Obtained from a Compounding Pharmacy

1. Testosterone Cream or Gel, 0.2%: Use a gel for the underside of the wrist or on the labia; use a cream to the vagina. Use 2 mg daily to begin with.

OR

2. Oral Micronized Testosterone, 2.5 mg: Take orally twice a day.

3. Use this amount for three months. Then re-assess your improvement and check your free testosterone levels. Most women will find 2–5 mg of testosterone cream or gel is the appropriate level; or 2.5–5 mg(twice a day) of the oral supplement.

No matter which preparation you use, assessment of your progress, symptoms, and possible side effects, as well as blood levels, should be done frequently, initially at 3-month intervals. Doses should be adjusted accordingly based on your results.

DON'T FORGET ABOUT VAGINAL DRYNESS

Painful intercourse for any reason, i.e. vaginal dryness due to decreased lubrication and thinning vaginal walls from decreased estrogen stimulation, is a common and well-known condition that affects most women at the perimenopause and menopause time. Specific attention to this problem, known as vaginal atrophy, is important. This can be a very significant contributor to your sexual issues at menopause. Details of therapies for vaginal atrophy were discussed at length in the previous chapter (Chapter 8).

MEDICINES TO ENHANCE SEXUAL DESIRE AND SEXUAL FUNCTION

Some of my patients prefer to take a medicine or herb before trying hormones. While there are no specific medicines/pharmacologic agents on the market to enhance libido or sexual function, some medicines seem to have some positive effects on female sexual function.

WELLBUTRIN® (BUPROPION) MAY HELP

The mild mood stabilizer and antidepressant Wellbutrin (bupropion) has been shown to increase general energy, sexual energy, desire, and even improve orgasms in some women. It is not specifically approved for these functions, but its potential for improvement of sexual function is widely accepted. If you have some depression, and are looking for an appropriate mild antidepressant that probably won't interfere with your sexual function, Wellbutrin might be an excellent choice.

The antidepressants in the SSRI family are known to decrease sexual desire and orgasms. If you are already taking an SSRI (selective serotonin reuptake inhibitor—mood stabilizer—antidepressant) for decreased mood, switching to or adding Wellbutrin and decreasing the amount of the SSRI may improve your sexual function.

BETTER SEX NATURALLY: LIBIDO BOOSTING HERBS AND OTHER SUBSTANCES

Many of my patients know that I am a chemist and natural therapist as well as a gynecologist, and that I have a large working knowledge of and recommend using herbs and natural therapies. Many women (as well as men) ask my advice for supplements which can boost their libido and sexual function. Since recorded time, healers have recommended and prescribed herbs and other substances as boosters of libido and sexual function. There has always been a search for the perfect aphrodisiac. When the relationship is good, and the medical situation is stable, there are a variety of natural substances that may boost your libido and intimate experiences.

Figure 9–2 outlines details about which herbs can be used safely for improved sexual function. Figure 9–3 explains herbs that probably won't work, and Figure 9–4 shows herbs and substances that may have serious side effects.

Figure 9–2

Better Sex Naturally: Herbs that Work

Herb	Proposed Function	Dose	When Not To Use
Gingko Biloba	• Improves blood flow • Increases intensity of orgasms • Improves erections in men	120 mg twice daily and an extra 120 mg 1 hour before intimacy	
Siberian Ginseng	• Improves sexual function by increasing testosterone levels	100–200 mg per day	If you have heart or kidney disease or high blood pressure, do not combine with prescription medicines without consulting your provider
Avena Satiua	• Improves low libido by increasing testosterone levels	300 mg per day	
Muira Puama	• Improves libido; improves male erections	1–1.5 gm per day	
Red Clover	• Improves blood flow	40 mg red clover isoflavones	
Maca Root	• Improves libido	3,000 mg daily	
St. John's Wort	• Decreases depression	300 mg three times per day	Do not take with SSRIs
L-Arginine	• An amino acid, not an herb, but it is natural; increases blood flow to the genitals	1,000 to 3,000 mg/day	Do not take if you suffer from migraines, autoimmune disorders, or herpes
Yohimbe	• Dilates blood vessels; may improve nerve function in the lower region of the spinal cord		• Can have side effects (See Figure 9–4); • Consult your medical provider before using

Do not take any of these herbs if you are pregnant, trying to conceive, or are on blood thinners.

Remember, herbs and other natural substances may be extremely useful and may have fewer potential side effects than pharmaceuticals. However,

Figure 9–3

Better Sex, Naturally: Herbs that Probably Won't Work

Herb	Proposed Function
Damiana	• Erectile enhancer in men and women • No research to support usefulness
Ashwagandha	• Increased potency, enhanced libido • No research: Folklore only
Wild Yam	• No research to support a wide variety of claims
Sarsparilla	• Impotence remedy in Latin America. • No research to support claims
Dong Quai	• Used in mixtures by Chinese herbalists. • No evidence for usefulness
Chasteberry (Vitex)	• Used by monks in early centuries. So named because it decreased libido in the monks

Do not take any of these herbs if you are pregnant, trying to conceive, or are on blood thinners.

choosing the right one is extremely important, and some knowledge about these herbs is critical to the decision. There are some herbs that may be useful, but some have potential side effects (for example, Yohimbe), and should be used with caution. Other herbs which are unsafe and dangerous should not be used at all.

It is also important to keep in mind that there are always questionable marketing practices and promotional articles produced surrounding herbs and natural substances. Use the information in this chapter as a guide, and always keep in mind that a reputable practitioner's help is very important.

More and more research shows that certain herbs may be at least moderately helpful for improving libido and sexual function. It is important to recognize that this research is in its infancy, and most data on herbs are not yet backed by rigorous, scientific-based evidence typically found with mainstream drugs. Long-term **traditional** use of many natural therapies suggest that many are likely safe, and possibly beneficial, in dealing with sexual problems. Keep in mind that, unlike stronger pharmaceuticals, **herbs usually need to be used for several weeks before results are seen.**

Herbs can cause interactions with other medications. If you are on other medications, check this out with your medical provider prescribing the other medications. Remember to check the purity and reliability of the specific brand of herb or supplement with www.ConsumerLab.com.

Figure 9–4

Better Sex, Naturally: Herbs That May Have SERIOUS Side Effects

Herb	Proposed Function	Side Effect
Yohimbe	• Increases blood flow and increases erections	• Can induce anxiety, increase heart rate, elevate blood pressure, cause flushing, headaches, and even hallucinations • Can be risky
Bee Pollen/Royal Jelly	• Folklore	• Literature documents asthma attacks, severe allergic reactions, and death • **UNSAFE & DANGEROUS!**
Spanish Fly	• Folklore • No data to support usefulness	• Can cause severe abdominal pain, burning of the mouth, vomiting, bleeding, and painful urination • **UNSAFE & DANGEROUS!**

Do not take any of these herbs if you are pregnant, trying to conceive, or are on blood thinners.

MY RECOMMENDATIONS: THE PERFECT MENOPAUSE NATURAL SEXUAL ENHANCEMENT FORMULA

The following combination of herbs and natural substances (Figure 9–5) is very useful and has been effective for my patients. Consider using this combination for 3 to 4 months, and see if you notice a difference. Refer back to Figure 9–2 for the function that each of these herbs performs. Some of these herbs may already be a part of your daily regimen if you've started therapy with "The Perfect Menopause Natural Therapy Formula" described in Chapter 6. I recommend starting with one supplement, and adding one supplement at a time every week until you are taking them all.

Figure 9–5

The Perfect Menopause Natural Sexual Enhancement Formula

Herb	Amount	Dosing Schedule
L-Arginine	1000–3000 mg	Once per day
Gingko Biloba	120 mg	2 times per day (add another 120 mg dose about 1 hour before intimacy)
Siberian Ginseng	500 mg	2 times per day, once in the morning, once at dinner. Do not take later in the evening as it may keep you awake.
Maca Root	3000 mg	Once per day
Red Clover	40 mg	Once per day
St. John's Wort	300 mg	3 times per day

Do not give up on this formula until at least 3 months of continuous use.

2. Decreased Blood Flow To The Genitals Due to Aging

Decreased blood flow to the genitals due to aging is a very real phenomenon that happens to every man and woman. **However, the number one treatment for decreased blood flow to the female genitals is the continuation of an active and stimulating sex life.** Yes, it's true! All you have to do is to continue to have a fulfilling and stimulating physical sex life, and this will stimulate improved blood flow to the genitals. For men, Viagra® and other erectile dysfunction medications improve blood flow. Unfortunately, it's not that simple for women. While the occasional woman responds to Viagra, it is usually ineffective.

However, there are things you **can** do to improve your blood flow in addition to the herbs and supplements in the Natural Sexual Enhancement Formula. These other things are very valuable when it comes to improving your intimate and sexual life as you age.

1. **Exercise.** Exercise increases blood flow in general, including to the genitals. Women (and men) who exercise, have greater genital blood flow than those who do not. Evidence shows that exercise improves your sex life!

2. **Good nutrition.** It should be obvious that good nutrition will improve blood flow. Controlling cholesterol and fats reduces negative cardiovascular effects, and improves blood flow. There are books written (example, *The Sex Diet*) on how a good diet improves sexual function.

3. **Hormones.** It is well known that estrogen improves blood flow to the genitals in women. Even small amounts of vaginal creams or other vaginal estrogens can make a big difference (see Chapter 8).

4. **Herbs.** As previously described in this chapter, several herbs are reported to improve blood flow to the genitals. The amino acid L-arginine, Gingko biloba, ginseng, red clover leaf, and yohimbe all improve blood flow.

Make every effort to improve your blood flow. It has a direct effect on your intimate life.

3. Medicines May Decrease Your Sexual Desire and Function

Many medications can cause decreased sexual desire and function. I am surprised by the number of women who do not know this, and who are prescribed medications without being told about the potential sexual side effects. The average woman who is 65 years of age will be taking at least seven medications, and one or more of them are very likely to affect sexual function.

One of the most frequently used medications that can cause a decreased libido and decreased orgasmic response are the SSRI antidepressants. If you take one of these medicines and are experiencing decreased desire and/or decreased orgasms, it is very likely playing a major role.

Other common medications that can cause a decrease in desire and/or orgasm are listed in Figure 9–6. If you or your partner are taking any one of these medicines and are experiencing sexual dysfunction, you should discuss this with your medical provider and consider an alternative therapy.

Figure 9–6

Drugs That Affect Sexuality In Women

	Decreased Desire	Diminished Arousal	Orgasmic Dysfunction
Anticholesterol medications	✓		
Antipsychotics	✓		✓
Barbituates	✓		
Benzodiazepines (ie, Valium®, Ambien®)	✓	✓	✓
Beta Blockers	✓		
Danazol	✓		
Digoxin	✓		
All SSRIs	✓	✓	✓
Gonadotropin Releasing Hormone Agonists	✓		
H₂ Blockers and Anti-Reflux Agents	✓		
Indomethacin	✓		
Ketoconazole	✓		
Lithium	✓		
Phenytoin	✓		
Spironolactone	✓		
Tricyclic Antidepressants	✓	✓	✓
Alcohol		✓	
Anticholinergics		✓	
Antihypertensives		✓	
Monoamine Oxidase Inhibitors		✓	
Aldomet			✓
Amphetemines and related Anorexia Drugs			✓
Narcotics			✓
Trazodone			✓
Birth Control Pills	✓	✓	✓
Oral Estrogens	✓	✓	✓

4. Some Medical Conditions Can Affect Your Sexual Function

There are acute and chronic medical conditions that can cause a significant decrease in desire and increase your difficulty achieving orgasm. For example, depression, high blood pressure, diabetes, increased cholesterol level, being overweight, and being a smoker can all have negative effects on your libido or ability to have orgasms. As long as other health issues are stable, sexual dysfunction usually improves in response to successful treatment of the medical condition (provided the therapy itself doesn't interfere). You should discuss all of your medical conditions with your menopause provider and let her/him know of your sexual dysfunction.

5 and 6. Identify and Fix a Stale Relationship and/or a Stale Sexual Relationship

A stale emotional relationship and/or a stale sexual relationship is one of the most significant causes of female sexual dysfunction at any age!

Look at Joan's situation:

Joan is a 72-year-old woman whose first husband died when she was 47. She has not really had a personal relationship with a man until last year when she met and fell in love with Dan, who is about her age. They are getting married in a few months. "You can't imagine," she told me, "the intense desire and passion that I have for Dan, even though we are waiting to be married before we are intimate." Joan told me she didn't recall having that much passion and intimacy for her first husband. It is likely that she did however, at least in the beginning of the relationship.

As we get older and live longer, many of us lose a partner either to death or to separation and divorce. Most of my patients who have lost their significant other, regardless of their age, find new relationships, and they become intense and passionate. This is a very important concept for a woman to understand about her sexual desire. New relationships can be intense, passionate, and very fulfilling. **An older, longer-term relationship can get stale!** A stale emotional and/or intimate relationship is frequently overlooked and not recognized as a cause of decreased sexual fulfillment, especially by women in midlife. **It's easy to blame hormones.**

Initially, when a couple is first together, their feelings and passion for each other are intense. They can't be away from each other and they frequently can't keep their hands off each other. A strong drive toward intimacy is beautiful and overwhelms all other aspects of life.

As time goes on, the realities and problems of life become more dominant in the relationship. Obligations, demands, and stresses of jobs, children, and other day-to-day issues overwhelm relationships. Job and career issues take time and energy, and when children come along, attention is diverted to them. In many instances, there is not enough time and not enough intimacy to keep the fires burning. The man and woman gravitate into specific roles in the relationship, and there is less time for each other. Some couples begin to grow apart.

The long-term nature of a sexual relationship begins to take over. The man is usually more easily aroused, and by nature, is more goal-oriented to the exact and specific act of intercourse. In general, desire is not so much of a problem for the man. A less intense personal relationship does not usually detract from a man's sexual desire.

The woman, however, is very different. A decrease in the warm emotional relationship diminishes her feelings of intimacy and sexual desire. This is the most common consequence in today's busy, overscheduled lifestyle, and the most common cause of decreased libido or sexual desire in my patients.

When women remain in a state of decreased sexual desire, this often leads to greater emotional disconnect, and the relationship often gets stale. The personal relationship between the couple begins to disintegrate, which can lead to separation and even divorce.

Has your relationship become stale? It may be worth considering that possibility.

Fix a Stale Relationship, or Find a New One?

If this sounds drastic or dramatic, I mean it to be. You really must look carefully at your relationship.

First, it is important to diagnose a stale relationship. Once diagnosed, you can begin the sometimes difficult but often rewarding work of rekindling your relationship. Doing this requires good communication, and it may require professional counseling. There are lots of subtle hurts, familiarities, and lost opportunities that will likely emerge in the process.

It could be worth it. A rejuvenated, intense personal relationship can bring the couple much joy and happiness. It's the source of great healing, and strong passion for each other spills over into all aspects of life.

This is the time to take a moment and look ahead. Close your eyes for a few minutes and fantasize—what would it be like if you had a rekindled passionate relationship with your partner? Can you envision it? Can you turn this around? Or do you only see intense passion happening with someone else?

Ask yourself at this point, "Is this the relationship I want for the rest of my life?" What can I do to stoke the fires of my stale relationship? An active, stimulating and passionate relationship, like a fire, requires daily feeding and stoking. It can only be as hot and sustained as what you put into it. Lack of attention is the culprit!

This Is a Major Issue and Requires an Honest Assessment and Difficult Decisions

A relationship is a partnership. If you don't give him attention, perhaps someone else will. And if he doesn't give you attention, you are not reaching your fantasy and fulfillment. Fixing a stale relationship may require professional help and counseling. If it is the right relationship though, then the efforts will be worth it a hundred times over. It is my feeling that most of us can use counseling at many points in our life, and the results will be worth it beyond imagination. This is one of those times.

REKINDLE A STALE SEXUAL RELATIONSHIP

If you are going to rekindle a stale sexual relationship, here is the number one guiding principle:

> For the woman, arousal comes before desire.
> For the man, desire comes before arousal.

This is a very important principle for both the man and the woman to understand. And this is especially important as a relationship progresses beyond the point when passion is automatic. As the relationship progresses, the passion that flows is the passion that the couple creates.

The man and woman must understand that the woman must be aroused before the desire/libido will develop. If couples really understood this, sexual desire or libido issues would be significantly reduced.

For both the woman and especially the man, the understanding that on a day-to-day basis, romancing—**arousing** the woman—during the day, and especially closer to the time of physical intimacy, will result in much more desire on her part. A woman wants to have her neck massaged. She wants a hug. Compliments and compassion come first. In a sense, a woman wants attention (foreplay) all day. She wants all-day niceties that lead her to want sex. And this is a circle. The more successful her all-day foreplay is, the more successful it will continue to be.

MAGAZINES/BOOKS/VIDEOS

You both must continue to be resourceful. Learning new ways to keep your intimate relationship fresh is extremely important. There are many magazines and good books on this topic. I used to find the stimulating sexual headlines on magazines such as *Cosmopolitan* or *Redbook* offensive, but as I began to read these articles, I recognized that they play an important role in keeping things fresh and imaginative in your intimate life. Keep an eye open for these articles and read them! As you continue to stimulate your relationship, these articles will motivate you to find new ways to keep your relationship fresh.

Another way to add new stimulation to your relationship, and therefore **desire,** is to consider instructional videos. There are several on the market today that are professionally made and tasteful, not vulgar. One example is *The Better Sex Video Series: Sexplorations* at BetterSex.com (or 1–800–955–0888). It is a very professionally done series, and many of my patients have found them useful. Watching these videos as a couple can offer a new dimension to your lovemaking, and can help keep subsequent passion and desire at high levels.

Resources for You

While I strongly recommend professional relationship counseling for this, here are four resources that you can begin with:

1. *Ultimate Relationship Program* is a DVD program by Anthony Robbins and Dr. Cloé Madanes (robbinsmadanes.com). It is a tremendous resource if you and your partner are looking to rekindle a stale relationship. It gives you steps to follow and case examples are reviewed and discussed. A straightforward, no-nonsense path for decisions and results is laid out for you to follow. I highly recommend this program.
2. *Passion Project* (www.loversforlife-media.com) is an extremely compelling program by Anthony and Sage Robbins on "what creates lasting passion." This newly released, 12-part series features several relationship experts focusing on the essentials of maintaining a lasting passionate and meaningful relationship.
3. *His Needs, Her Needs—Building An Affair-Proof Marriage* by William F. Harley, Jr. This is an outstanding book which asks the question, "Do you know your own marital needs? Do you know the marital needs of your spouse?" I strongly recommend this book.

4. *Making Love The Way We Used To—Or Better: Secrets To Satisfying Midlife Sexuality* by Alan M. Altman, M.D. and Laurie Ashner. This timely book looks at the intimacy issues of the midlife woman, and complements what you have read in this book.

DO YOU NEED A NEW RELATIONSHIP?

Be honest and frank with yourself. Don't keep things the way they are if they are not the way you want them. Perhaps it's plain and simple that this is not the right relationship for you no matter how long you've been together or how old you are. You and your mate's life goals may have become different over time and you may be headed in different directions and with different interests. Life is short! Change can be hard, but it can be worth it. If this is not the right relationship, this may be the time to make that decision. **You may need counseling to help you make this decision, but at least make the decision to get counseling**.

Rekindling a stale relationship or building a new one can be a tremendous asset to a sagging libido at menopause. Remember my patient Joan. Her new, beautiful relationship at 72 years old is not unusual! Her passion spreads to her entire life. It is contagious.

7. Communication

Finding new and fresh ways for you and your partner to not only communicate, but to stimulate each other, is the key ingredient to making any of these sexual enhancements work. Communication can keep the intimacy progressing forward, and the intimacy that results will keep the communication going. Some of the causes of decreased sexuality will require time and patience to overcome, and being able to talk about your issues, feelings, and progress with your partner can make a huge difference in your success. Remember, an intimate relationship is an intimate communication between the two of you. You must have a special relationship with each other. Communicate! **Communicate!**

Bonus: An Intimate and Passionate Relationship Eases Your Other Menopause Symptoms

There is probably nothing better or more healing in life than a beautiful and fulfilling personal, intimate, and passionate relationship. When this exists, **desire abounds.** With an intense intimate and passionate relationship, endorphins in your body flow, and these endorphins soothe and reduce all of your other menopause symptoms. And as you might guess, all your other health issues are improved also.

DRAMATICALLY IMPROVE YOUR SEXUAL DESIRE

In Step 6, we have covered a wide variety of issues that can impact your sexual satisfaction. You owe it to yourself and your partner to really assess all of these issues carefully. Feeling sexually fulfilled need not be a thing of your past, however you will need to take action to reclaim your sexuality. If you are committed to it, you will certainly succeed in dramatically improving your sexual desire.

Take action today on what you have learned in this chapter.
You will be rewarded more than one hundred fold.

Maybe all that is getting between you and a great sex life is the lack of a good night's sleep. In that case, Step 7 addresses how you can improve your sleep, and help you to feel rested and rejuvenated. Whether it is your intimate life, social life, or family life that suffers, get ready to banish the "I'm too tired!" excuse!

BEFORE WE DISCUSS SLEEP

Before we discuss the importance of a good night's sleep, let's look at one more thing that could be a factor in your sexual desire, and that is **the sexual desire of your mate.**

DOES YOUR MATE HAVE MALE MENOPAUSE?
IS THERE A MALE MENOPAUSE?

You bet there is! Most men don't recognize male menopause in themselves, but you will notice it, and you can help him through it.

For years, scientists have studied and written about the male climacteric or **male menopause**. The thinking is that middle aged men often experience some of the same physical and emotional problems as women in midlife. In the extreme, these changes can make a man desperate to recapture his youth.

In men, hormones may not play as significant a role in this midlife crisis as it does for women. Men have smaller amounts of estrogen than women and this often slightly increases with age, rather than the decrease noted in women. Men have high levels of testosterone, and as it does in women, this slowly declines with age. Men generally lose 0.5% of testosterone annually beginning at age 40, but their testosterone rarely gets below healthy levels. When a man's testosterone does dramatically decline, this is different from the normal male menopause, and is known as **andropause**. Women can suffer andropause also. But andropause is not what we mean by "male menopause."

For many men, the early signs of male menopause may only be noticeable to a partner: a decrease in libido, sour moods, lack of motivation or energy, or a blend of fatigue and anxiety, increasing difficulty with sleep, depression, muscle and bone loss, and abdominal weight gain. Some men even verbalize concerns about aging and mortality.

While male menopause can begin anywhere between ages 40 to 70, it usually begins around age 50, the same age as the female menopause. Its cause, however, is different. Male menopause is more frequently associated with the now recognizable, cumulative effects of many years of bad lifestyles, habits, and stress. Affection for smoking, sofas, decreased exercise, poor eating, environmental exposures, and occupational stresses are highly associated with male menopause and rapid aging.

For women, hot flashes frequently signal the beginning of menopause or perimenopause. Men usually first notice symptoms of male menopause when their ability to achieve or sustain an erection begins to wane. While this is a very common problem, and medical treatment is widely available, many men still do not seek the treatment because of the reluctance to discuss the problem. A common reaction from the woman is to take the blame herself, and to begin to doubt her femininity, especially at this very sensitive time in her life.

TREATMENTS ARE AVAILABLE FOR MALE MENOPAUSE

Often, changes in lifestyle can reverse the problems of male menopause. **However, the first course of action is to make sure that the symptoms are not the first signs of andropause.** If his symptoms begin before age 45, or his symptoms are extreme, these can be early signs of "hypogonadism" or andropause, and these possibilities need to be evaluated. Evaluation of hormone levels—including testosterone (total and free), DHEA, estradiol, thyroid, and even cortisol—is very appropriate. Bioidentical hormone therapies would be appropriate if these levels are too low. I strongly encourage that the differential diagnosis between male menopause and andropause be made before an appropriate course of therapies is decided.

If his symptoms turn out to be male menopause and not andropause, you can help him with lifestyle changes. All men will experience some male menopause symptoms as they age. For most men, the degree of their symptoms will depend on their general health and the degree to which they take action and modify their lifestyle.

7 STEPS FOR YOU TO HELP HIM TO ACHIEVE THE PERFECT MALE MENOPAUSE

1. **Stop smoking.** Nicotine may increase the formation of blockages in the vessels that supply blood to all the organs, including the penis. Studies have shown some men will get firmer erections when they stop smoking. In addition to this practical issue, increased blood flow to all organs will increase vitality, general health, and longevity.

2. **A low-fat diet.** Changing to a low-fat diet will help him slow down aging in general, as well as improve blood flow to the penis. Foods that are good for the heart are good for the penis also, since the smaller blood vessels of the penis often become clogged before those of the heart.

3. **Manage medication.** Virtually any medication can cause some form of impotence. Antidepressants and high blood pressure medications have the worst track records. If sexual dysfunction is a major component of his male menopause, ask his provider to change his medication to reduce side effects.

4. **Manage depression.** Recognize that stress and depression are common in men in this age group, and that stress and depression can decrease overall well-being, as well as sexual desire and function. Acknowledge and deal with his job stress, family stress, financial stress, and marriage and relationship issues. Management of these problems will also have a tremendous value in the management of your menopause, your relationship, and your health and vitality.

5. **Exercise.** Most men begin to lose significant muscle mass beginning around age 40. As much as 1% of muscle mass per year is lost unless a significant and active exercise program is maintained. There are many other benefits to maintaining a regular exercise program. Relative to male menopause, exercise improves mental clarity as well as overall well-being, and increases blood flow (including to the penis), all of which are very necessary components to maintaining a healthy sexual function.

6. **Get regular medical checkups, including a midlife physical exam.** Men are not as compulsive as women in seeing their health care providers for what they deem as "little problems." Consequently, medical situations that begin as small problems can grow into significant problems before they are recognized. Examples include hypertension, heart disease, and a diseased prostate. Schedule him for a midlife comprehensive physical exam with his health-care provider, and then make sure that he has regular checkups as appropriate.

7. **Use appropriate vitamins and supplements.** Men as well as women can benefit from supplements that can improve health, vigor and vitality. This is even more important at the time of the male menopause.

Specific vitamins and supplements will depend upon his medical situation. However, in general, I recommend consideration of one or more of the following:

- **A daily multivitamin**
- **Fish oils or flaxseed oil—1000 mg twice a day,** for cardiovascular health
- **Gingko biloba—120 mg twice a day** for improved cognition, and improved blood flow to the genitals. An extra 120 mg prior to intimacy may also be helpful for improved blood flow
- **L-Arginine—1000 to 3000 mg a day** for improved blood flow/ increased erections
- **Siberian ginseng—500 mg one to two times a day** for increased energy, increased metabolism, and improvement in sexual function (Do not take ginseng after supper, as it may prevent a restful sleep.)
- **Saw palmetto—320 mg a day** to help reduce prostate swelling, improve urination control, and improve sexual function
- **Maca root—2000 to 3000 mg once per day** to improve mental and physical energy, focus, and sexual function
- Other herbs and vitamins can be added to this list, depending on his needs and medical situation

Assess his male menopause now, and make a decision to do something about it. Don't put it off. Management of his male menopause will complement your therapies for your menopause, and make your menopause transition easier. Ask him to do what I have asked you to do in this book. Ask him to look at himself in the mirror, and recognize how much he has changed in the last five years. Then ask him to look forward and estimate how he will look five years from now! Develop a plan. You can prevent many aspects of aging, both in yourself and him. But you must take action now! Just as you can have The Perfect Menopause, he too can have The Perfect Male Menopause.

chapter 10

Step Seven
You Can Have A
Better Night's Sleep

Are You Tired of Being Tired?
Have You Given Up On a Good Night's Sleep?

POOR SLEEP IS ONE OF THE MOST common complaints of women at the time of menopause. In my practice, I would rank it as the third most common complaint, following weight gain and decreased sexual desire. Some of my patients have trouble falling asleep. But the majority of them fall asleep, wake up one or more times during the night, and then have difficulty getting back to sleep. Does this sound like you?

HOW DOES POOR SLEEP AFFECT YOU?

Poor sleep will affect how you feel overall. If you don't sleep well, you may experience more depressed moods, increased anxiety, decreased daytime energy, and greater difficulty with thinking and focusing. A recent study has even linked weight gain with fewer than 7.7 hours of sleep per night. A decreased interest in sex, a decreased interest in overall productivity, poorer health and less happiness may also be attributed to inferior sleeping. In short, poor sleep exacerbates many of the menopausal symptoms you may already be experiencing!

WHY IS SLEEP SO DIFFICULT FOR YOU?

We really don't know why sleep is so difficult for women at menopause. There are several theories, but studies are inconclusive. Here is what we do know:

1. **Hormones**. Studies looking at hormones and sleep show that there is a relationship, but exactly how hormones affect sleep has not yet been figured out. It has been shown in a clinical setting that women taking either estrogen or progesterone do sleep better, both in how long and how deeply they sleep.

2. **Age.** There are many studies showing that we sleep less effectively as we age. Again, exact mechanisms are not clearly understood.

3. **Stress**. Stress is known to cause sleep dysfunction by increasing cortisol levels. Cortisol, familiarly known as adrenalin, puts us into an immediate energy mode, which obviously serves to stimulate, rather than relax us.

4. **Poor lifestyles**. Poor nutrition, inadequate exercise, smoking, using too much alcohol or caffeine, and even a poor sleep environment (such as having a TV on in your bedroom) have all been shown in numerous studies to contribute to poor sleep.

5. **Increased tendency toward sleep apnea**. An increase in neck size increases your risk for sleep apnea. There are lots of theories for this, including hormonal changes as well as weight gain.

6. **Increased weight.** Increased weight at menopause has been linked with insomnia. This may be due to increased cortisol levels, or to an increased tendency toward sleep apnea, or both.

7. **Chronic health issues**. Chronic diseases such as diabetes, hypertension, anxiety, depression, hyperthyroidism, asthma, and many other significant health issues are known to interfere with sleep.

8. **Side effects from both prescription and over-the-counter medicines.** Many medications have stimulating effects. For example, the antidepressant Wellbutrin works on the dopamine neurotransmitter system. If taken at night, it will stimulate rather than relax you, and you won't sleep well. Similarly, many supplements contain caffeine, which interferes with sleep. The herb ginseng will keep you awake if you take it late in the day.

The self-questionnaire in Figure 10–1 is designed to help you consider the possible reasons for your poor sleep. Answer the questions, and use your answers to help find solutions. There are many reasons for sleep dysfunction, and your answers to these questions will help point you to your possible culprit. Make a copy of this questionnaire with your answers, and share it with your menopause provider.

Figure 10–1

Questionnaire About Sleep and Sleepiness

- How have you been sleeping recently?
- If you have a sleep problem, is it associated with significant fatigue or a noticeable decline in productivity or concentration the next day? How bothersome is it?
- When did the problem begin? (Is it acute or chronic insomnia?)
- How often do you experience hot flashes/sweats during the day and night?
- Do you experience frequent nighttime awakenings, and can you go back to sleep easily?
- Do you have early morning awakenings and daytime fatigue?
- Do you have a psychiatric or medical condition that may cause insomnia, such as depression, anxiety, hyperthyroidism, excess caffeine intake, or are you taking any medications?
- Is your sleep environment conducive to sleeping?
- Do you experience "creeping," "crawling," or other uncomfortable feelings in your legs that are relieved by moving the legs?
- Do you snore loudly, gasp, choke or stop breathing during sleep?
- Do you have morning symptoms such as increased nasal congestion, dry mouth, and headache?
- What are your bedtimes and rise times on weekdays and weekends?
- Do you use caffeine, tobacco or alcohol? Do you take over-the-counter or prescription medications (such as stimulating antidepressants, steroids, decongestants, or beta blockers)?
- How high is your general stress level now? What are some of your major stresses? Are they limited or ongoing? Does anxiety seem to be a component of why you are waking up or can't go back to sleep?

SOLUTIONS TO YOUR SLEEP PROBLEMS

No matter what the cause, there are solutions that will work for you!

As I have done in other areas of this book, I am describing solutions to your sleep problems under three broad categories: natural therapies, medicinal or pharmaceutical therapies, and hormone therapies.

NATURAL THERAPIES

Natural therapies for insomnia are often very successful, and I strongly recommend that you try them first for your sleep problems. If you are patient and persistent, there is a significant chance that they will work for you. Natural therapies that work include:

- **Lifestyle changes.** Lifestyle changes are very important in managing your sleep difficulties. The major lifestyle changes that will work can be found in Figure 10–2. Make the decision today to make lifestyle changes that will improve not only your sleep, but your overall health and happiness.

Figure 10–2

Lifestyle Issues

- Get to, and maintain, a healthy weight.
- Discontinue caffeine intake 4 to 6 hours before bedtime and minimize total daily use.
- Avoid nicotine, especially near bedtime or during nighttime awakenings.
- Avoid the use of alcohol in the late evening.
- Eat meals on a regular schedule. Eat a light snack (but not a heavy meal) before bedtime if you are hungry.
- Get regular exposure to outdoor sunlight, especially in the late afternoon.

- **Sleep hygiene.** Over time, improvement in your sleep hygiene will also improve the quality of your sleep. Figure 10–3 provides a variety of sleep hygiene changes you ought to consider trying. If these changes in sleep hygiene seem to help, consider reading a book on feng shui. These

Figure 10–3

Sleep Hygiene

- Keep regular bedtimes and wake times, even on weekdays and days off from work.
- Limit total time in bed to 8 hours.
- Avoid daytime naps. If you must nap, do so early in the afternoon and for no longer than 30 minutes per day.
- Establish a bedtime routine and do the same thing every night before you go to bed. For example, take a warm (not hot) bath and then read for 10 minutes every night before going to bed.
- Use the bedroom only for sleeping and having sex. Don't eat, talk on the telephone, or watch television while you are in bed.
- Minimize noise, light and excessive temperatures during the sleep period. If noise is a problem, use a fan to cover the noise or use earplugs.
- Move the alarm clock away from the bed if it is a source of distraction or worry.
- If you're still awake after trying to fall asleep for 30 minutes, get up and go to another room. Sit quietly for 20 minutes, and then go back to bed. Do this as many times as you need to until you fall asleep.

concepts are designed to improve harmony in your life by creating harmony in your surroundings, which will improve your sleep.

- **Meditation/hypnosis.** Meditation and/or self hypnosis are powerful natural therapies to improve your sleep. I have used meditation and self hypnosis personally for many years, and find them satisfying, peaceful, and invigorating. Meditation and self hypnosis CDs are easy to find in bookstores or on the Internet. One of my favorites is *Mindful Meditation* by Jon Kabat-Zinn, Ph.D. Dr. Kabat-Zinn is an expert in mindful meditation, and his CD program is a masterpiece. If you get this program and use it 20 minutes a day (or even every other day) you will tremendously benefit from it. It can be ordered from Nightingale Conant (1–800–525–9000) or at www.nightingale.com. I recommend this program first. Other favorites of mine include: *Hypnology* by Dick Sulphen (also available at Nightingale Conant), *The Ultimate Brain* by Tom Kenyon, M.A. (www.tomkenyon.com), and *Heal Yourself with Medical Meditation* by Drs. Andrew Weil and Steven Gungevich (1–800–3DR-WEIL). Try one of these programs.

They can help you enjoy a more relaxed, healthful life, and you will sleep much better. And keep using them. A peaceful and relaxed mind will keep you sleeping well and provide a much healthier, happy life.

- **Herbs and natural substances**. There are many herbs and natural substances that can help in the management of your sleep. If you have one that works, and it is safe, keep using it. If you have never tried herbs or natural substances to help with sleep, you may be in for a pleasant surprise. I've kept track of the ones that have been the most useful for my patients over the years, and I recommend that you follow these guidelines:

  1. **Valerian root.** Valerian root is one of the most popular and effective herbs for sleep management. I strongly recommend that you try Valerian root first. If you try it for just a few nights, you won't notice an improvement. Like all herbs, you need to take it at bedtime every night for at least 3 months before it is really effective. Be patient, and Valerian root will help improve your sleep.
  2. **Passion flower and hops.** Passion flower and hops are herbs similar to Valerian root in their usefulness for improving sleep. While I have found Valerian root to be the most successful single herb for insomnia, a combination of Valerian root with Passion flower and/or hops produces even better sleep. General Nutrition Center (GNC) sells a product called "Sleep Formula," which is a combination of all of these herbs, and it is excellent. Many of my patients use this product very successfully. Remember to take it every night to maximize its effectiveness.
  3. **Magnesium.** Proper amounts of magnesium also aid in a restful night's sleep. Some of my patients take only magnesium and notice an improvement in their sleep. Magnesium can help your achy and/or restless legs also. For best results, magnesium should be taken with balanced amounts of calcium. Calcium magnesium citrate, or a preparation containing 500 mg of calcium citrate and 250 of magnesium citrate, is my recommendation. Both of these are also contained in the GNC preparation "Sleep Formula" mentioned above.

4. **Lavender.** Lavender is an essential oil that has calming effects, and is often mentioned as a sleeping aid. Although there are several forms on the market, including Lavender tea, most of them are minimally effective in helping with significant insomnia. Lavender may be useful as a spritz or pillow mist at bedtime, or even as an additive to your evening session in your bath tub. In this manner, it may be very relaxing. I use it myself in both of these ways.

5. **Melatonin.** Melatonin is a hormone that regulates your sleep/wake cycle and other daily biorhythms. There is considerable scientific data on melatonin, and it is thought to have a significant effect on your moods and circadian rhythms. It is thought that the body's production of melatonin is based on the day/night cycle. A good night's sleep in a dark room is important for adequate production of melatonin, as well as exposure to daytime sunlight, especially in the afternoon. If it has been a while since you have had a good night's sleep, then melatonin supplementation may be useful to help promote sleep.

　　Synthetic, bioidentical melatonin has recently become available as an over-the-counter supplement. For my patients, I have always found that Valerian root and the above-mentioned supplements work better than melatonin for sleep. But for some of my patients, melatonin has worked very well. I prefer the sublingual tablets, which dissolve under the tongue. The common dosage for occasional use is 2.5 to 3 mg. For regular use, 0.25 to 0.3 mg before bed is an effective dose. Some patients find that with regular use they have a "hangover" effect. If that happens to you, try the other herbs discussed above. If you are in a "sleep rut" and are going to start melatonin, try this formula: Start with 3 mg sublingual 1 hour before bed every night for one week, then step down your dose over the next two weeks until you reach 0.3 mg each night. Continue to use the 0.3 mg every night as a maintenance dose.

I urge you to use natural therapies first to try to resolve your sleep difficulties. They are safe, effective, and can be used long-term without any worries.

MEDICINES/PHARMACEUTICALS

For some of my patients, the insomnia problem is difficult enough to require medicinal therapies. Fortunately, there are two categories of medicinal therapies that are mild and effective for significant sleep dysfunction at menopause:

1. **Nonspecific medicines.** The same medications used to treat hot flashes, night sweats, and mood dysfunction may also be helpful to treat a sleep dysfunction. The SSRI medications, particularly Effexor, Paxil, Zoloft, and Prozac, may help alleviate anxiety, depression, and/or night sweats and help improve your sleep. Neurontin (gabapentin) may also be useful, but I have found it less effective for sleep issues. The same doses should be used as described in Chapter 6.

2. **Specific medicines.** There are newer, milder sleep medications that are very effective when natural therapies don't work. They can be especially useful in the short term, although some women find them necessary to use over the long term. These medications, including Ambien®, Lunesta®, and Rozerem®, are the latest developments in mild, short-acting, sleep medications, and may be effective and safe to use, even for several months when necessary.

   Ambien comes in 5 or 10 mg doses, Lunesta comes in 1, 2, and 3 mg doses, and Rozerem is available as an 8 mg dose. Patients differ in their experiences with each of these medicines. What works for one woman may work differently for another woman.

   In general, my patients seem to prefer Ambien. For many, a 5 mg dose, or even half of a 5 mg dose, works well. Occasionally, a patient will need 10 mg. If getting to sleep is your problem, it works best when you dissolve the pill under your tongue (sublingual). However, most women find that staying asleep is their biggest problem. In this case, swallowing the whole pill with a small amount of food helps to prolong the absorption, allowing Ambien to work better throughout the night.

   Ambien also makes a slow release product called Ambien CR. It comes in 6.25 mg and 12.5 mg doses. For many of my patients, Ambien CR causes some morning drowsiness. If that is the case for you, switch back to the regular Ambien, and take it with food as recommended above.

If you aren't sleeping well because of restless legs, there is a new medicine now available to help you. Requip® is specifically for restless legs, and if your restless legs are causing your difficult sleep, this medicine may help improve your sleep. If your restless legs are mild, simply taking 400 mg of magnesium every night at bedtime may work.

Sleep experts generally agree that natural therapies and behavioral changes, as well as the newer medicinal therapies, all work in the management of sleep dysfunction. However, sleep experts also acknowledge that it is difficult to get Americans to be patient with natural therapies and behavioral changes in the management of their sleep problems. If you need to take medicines for the short term, I urge you to work on incorporating natural therapies also for your longer-term sleep health.

NOTE: You have probably seen news bulletins recently about the side effects from some of these sleep medications, such as sleep walking, sleep driving, and sleep eating. Most people don't have these problems at *normal* doses. If you note any unusual side effects, report these immediately to your menopause provider.

HORMONE THERAPIES

Scientists are not sure why hormone therapies seem to work for sleep dysfunction for women at this time of perimenopause/menopause, but it is clear that they do work. Women who elect to take estrogen for other reasons almost always report a dramatic improvement in their sleep.

Estrogen therapy for sleep dysfunction usually only requires a very low dose of estrogen. Consistent with my recommendations in Chapters 5 and 6, when estrogen therapy is used, I prefer to start with a very low dose of transdermal bioidentical estradiol. Specific doses and regimens are discussed in Chapters 5 and 6.

Although progesterone has a natural sedative effect, I prefer not to use it specifically for sleep dysfunction. You will recall that there continues to be a controversy that progesterone, rather than estrogen, may be a factor in breast cancer. Frankly, there are too many other effective and safe alternatives available to justify the use of daily progesterone for sleep dysfunction.

YOU CAN HAVE A BETTER NIGHT'S SLEEP

In Step 7 we've explored some of the important principles of good sleep. The remarkable thing about sleep dysfunction is that this is one of the easier issues to resolve without having to see a doctor at all! There are so many little lifestyle changes you can implement, or great over-the-counter herbs and vitamins that you can take, to help you improve your sleep, and all you have to do is make the commitment to change your sleep habits.

Getting a better night's sleep is the last step of the *The Perfect Menopause: 7 Steps to the Best Time of Your Life*. However, there is one other important issue that I've brought up many times. Throughout this book, I've urged you to work with your menopause provider. You may have one that you already like and work well with, and that is great! If you don't, you might be asking, "How do I find this health care practitioner who will be my partner through my menopause years?" The next chapter will provide you with tips on how to find the perfect menopause provider for you. It will help you figure out what you need to look for, and how to interview a health care provider to determine if she/he is the right fit for you.

Chapter 11 will also provide tips on how you can best maximize your time with your menopause provider. It is important that you properly prepare for your appointments with your health care practitioner so that you can be sure to address all of your questions and get the answers and advice you are seeking. No matter where you are in your search for your menopause provider, the next chapter contains valuable information that everyone can benefit from.

PART**THREE**

More Resources to Help You Achieve a Perfect Menopause

chapter 11

How to Choose and Work with the Perfect Medical Provider

DO YOU WONDER HOW YOU CAN FIND a knowledgeable and caring medical provider who has an interest in your menopause? One of the most important people in the successful management of your menopause is the right medical care provider, one who can answer your questions and can help you find safe and effective solutions to your unique menopause.

The perfect menopause practitioner is caring, has the knowledge, training, experience, and the interest and time to offer you all the up-to-date options. The right practitioner can make the difference between having an average (or worse, miserable) menopause and making these years the best of your life.

THE BEST PRACTITIONER CHOICES

Your practitioner choice could be a physician or nurse practitioner and will most likely be trained in the area of OB/GYN, internal medicine, or family practice. Look for someone special. Remember, most doctors (even OB/GYNs) weren't rigorously trained about menopause. Even in the best OB/GYN residencies, menopause gets little formal attention, and many medical practices are simply too busy in today's HMO style of practice to pay proper attention to your menopause needs if it is not their special interest.

The good news is that times are changing. As more women reach the menopause age, more health care practitioners are becoming interested in menopause and menopause therapies. More and more practitioners are acquiring special knowledge and training to become experts in understanding and treating menopause. The North American Menopause Society (NAMS) is the largest national medical Society dedicated to menopause research and education. This highly respected organization credentials practitioners as menopause experts when they have met certain educational expectations, including special training and passing special exams in menopause management.

Menopause is your special time in life. Look for someone special: one who knows all the options and is open to them.

HOW TO FIND YOUR SPECIAL PRACTITIONER

Is someone special caring for you now? If it is your OB/GYN, are you getting enough attention? Your OB/GYN may be the perfect provider, but just may not be aware that you're interested in more time to discuss menopause options. Maybe your OB/GYN doesn't have the time or specific interest, but is willing to refer you to someone else in the practice or in the community who does have an interest and expertise in menopause.

Ask people in your community to find out who are the menopause experts. Look to your friends for some information. They may know or have had an experience with someone they have found very helpful. Your internist or family practitioner is a good resource also. And be sure to consult your pharmacist. She or he may know a great practitioner with a special interest in menopause. Also, consider making inquiries at the local medical society, with friends who are in the medical profession, at hospitals, medical centers and local medical schools.

As a few names filter out, first check their credibility online or check with friends who may have some input on the specific individuals. The North American Menopause Society is one place you will want to check for credentials. You can find a lot of up-to-date and accurate information in the consumer section of their website, where they manage a list of doctors and other health care practitioners who belong to this Society. The website can be found at: http://www.menopause.org/consumers/.

MAXIMIZE YOUR MEETING: THE PERFECT APPOINTMENT

Once you've made an appointment with the menopause practitioner, I strongly recommend that you carefully **prepare for this visit.** You are looking for a menopause practitioner who will spend the necessary time with you, and you will want to maximize this time. Advanced preparation will allow you to use your allotted time efficiently and effectively. I recommend the same preparation for each additional visit.

Ask that your first visit be a consultation, and ask the office staff how long it will last. At your first visit, I recommend covering these three agenda items:

1. Give the provider information about who you are, why you are there, and what specific interests you have.
2. Learn about the provider, the provider's knowledge, special training, interest and philosophies regarding menopause and menopause therapies, especially as it relates to you.
3. Learn how the practice works in relationship to your needs. Is the provider and practice the right one for you?

WHO YOU ARE!

The very first thing you want to do at your first visit is provide accurate, detailed information quickly and efficiently about who you are and why you are looking for a new provider. **Writing this information down beforehand, in a clear, concise, and brief manner, will help you focus and communicate your issues, questions and needs quickly and concisely.** Figure 11–1 contains a brief form that will help you summarize all of this information. Copy it, fill it out, and give a copy to the provider. This will save valuable time, and allow more time to be spent on important answers to your questions and counseling.

I also recommend that you document your visits and keep your notes organized. Keep a copy of the completed form and your personal notes from the visit in your new folder labeled with your practitioner's name on it.

Also at your first visit, let the practitioner know your philosophies about menopause, and what your initial thinking is about treatment options. (You

---

Figure 11–1

Simple Form For Your Practitioner

Fill out this form and give it to your new practitioner as a quick outline of your medical history.

NAME: _____ AGE: _____

Problem(s): (Why I came here) _____
(*Be concise*)
_____
_____

Medications: _____

Vitamins/Supplements: _____

I have had the following:

When:

☒   Mammogram   _____

☒   DEXA Bone Density   _____

☒   Colonoscopy   _____

☒   Cholesterol Testing _____

☒   Hormone Testing   _____

☒   Other Special Tests _____

should have a few ideas now that you have read *The Perfect Menopause: 7 Steps to the Best Time of Your Life* Acknowledge that you are open minded and looking for options. For example, "I was hoping to do this more naturally," or, "I was hoping to start on hormones." This will let the provider know the starting point. Write down the reasons for your visit in advance to help you prepare and focus better at the visit.

It is also very helpful if you let the provider know what you have been reading and hearing about. Not everything that is written is absolutely true or scientifically accurate. Some therapies may not be appropriate for you. Don't forget that our understanding and knowledge about menopause and menopause therapies are rapidly changing. Be sure to keep an open mind about your options for management, because as Professor Einstein said, "The answers have changed!"

LEARN ABOUT THE PROVIDER

Your second agenda point is to learn about the provider and to get specific feedback about how she/he can help you make menopause the best time of your life. You probably already know the practitioner's medical credentials but if you don't, ask! Ask about general and specific medical training, and with which hospital(s) she/he is affiliated. Find out who covers emergency calls when she/he is away or "not on call."

With regard to menopause, I recommend that you consider some or all of the following questions:

1. Do you have a special interest in menopause? What percent of your patients are in menopause and perimenopause?
2. Do you have special training or an expertise in the area of menopause? Where did you do your training?
3. Do you believe in, and treat patients when appropriate, with:
    a. Hormone therapies?
    b. Herbal therapies?
    c. Other natural therapies such as acupuncture, meditation, chiropractic, and hypnosis?

4. Are you open-minded with regard to working with other natural therapists such as naturopaths, herbalists, acupuncturists, and chiropractors?
5. Do you measure and evaluate hormone levels (serum and/or salivary),
   bone densities, cholesterol levels, mammograms, and colonoscopies as
   part of management?
6. Are you familiar with bioidentical hormones? Do you use them in your
   practice? Why or why not?
7. Do you recommend compounding pharmacies, pharmaceuticals, or
   both as sources for therapies?
8. Do you actively manage patients for sexual dysfunction? Mood
   dysfunction? Weight management? Cognitive dysfunction? Insomnia?
9. How would you begin to coach me about my menopause?
10. What would be the time frame to achieve this/these goals?
11. Where do we go from here?

IS THE PROVIDER RIGHT FOR YOU?

After the first visit, you should be able to decide if the provider is right for you
and your situation. If this is not the right provider for you, move on to your
next option. Don't waste time. If this is the right situation, begin to build a
solid relationship with the provider. Find out how the practice works, so that
you can communicate effectively with your practitioner, and follow-up as frequently as recommended. You will be on your way to making the menopause
years the best years of your life.

INSIDER TIPS TO MORE EFFECTIVE OFFICE VISITS

Even with the perfect menopause provider and a great start, achieving The
Perfect Menopause requires continuing forward momentum. Make each visit
to your practitioner effective and productive using these five tips:

1. **Take notes.** Bring a pad and pen to take notes, especially at consultations. Even if you write down only a few things, you can review them

when you get home and you will recall the issues more clearly. Don't waste the opportunity to put all the good advice from your visit into action. **You won't get results unless you take action.**

2. **Keep a menopause journal.** Journaling is a very effective way to help you take action. Daily entries would be best, but even weekly entries will help you reflect on your menopause issues, and monitor your progress. Write down what you plan to do in order to tackle your sleep dysfunction, weight gain, hot flashes, mood swings, sexual issues, or anything else you want to start changing, and keep a log of your provider's recommendations. Make notations about how many hot flashes you had that day, how you are feeling about your significant other, and anything else that will help you monitor your progress. Figure 11–3 is an example of a typical journal form for menopause. Bring your menopause journal or a summary of it with you to your office visits. And write down your questions in advance too, so you won't forget (Figure 11–2).

3. **Turn off your cell phone.** Nothing is more distracting (yet surprisingly common) as a patient, in the middle of a consultation with the practitioner, to get a cell phone call and even worse, actually answer it. Don't break the concentration! First impressions are very important for you as well as the practitioner. Golden Rule: do unto others as you would have them do unto you. If you want to get the most out of your consultation, be sure to respect the time and efforts of the practitioner. Build the partnership you want and maintain it in the best possible manner.

4. **Ask for recommended reading.** Ask the practitioner for references and reading recommendations. Read good, balanced literature and be open-minded about, yet critical of, the validity of what is being presented. Be aware that there is a great deal written about menopause and menopause therapy, and not all of it is accurate, balanced, or medically sound.

5. **Manage your insurance coverage.** Don't make payment for your consultations and visits an issue. As best as you are able, determine **in advance** what insurance(s) the provider participates in, what your insurance covers, and what your out-of-pocket responsibility will be. A busy menopause practitioner wants to take care of your medical issues, not spend considerable time collecting payments or figuring out your insurance. This is a frequent issue and big headache in many office

practices today. Don't let payments or insurance issues dilute an otherwise outstanding provider-patient relationship.

Take every opportunity to attain The Perfect Menopause, and make these the best years of your life. A big part of this will be finding the right menopause practitioner, and then working to establish an effective and ongoing relationship with that provider.

Figure 11–2

Questions to Ask the Provider

_____

_____

_____

_____

_____

_____

_____

_____

_____

_____

_____

_____

_____

_____

_____

_____

_____

_____

_____

_____

_____

_____

Figure 11–3

The Perfect Menopause Journal

chapter

12

Put Your Plan into Action: Make These the Best Years of Your Life

WHILE I HAVE PRACTICED ALL ASPECTS of obstetrics and gynecology, every day I see several menopause patients in my office. Most of them listen, and many of them will follow some of my advice. A few follow my advice completely and achieve outstanding success and improvement.

Many years ago, a patient who had achieved tremendous successes from our work together embroidered and framed my favorite poem, Robert Frost's "The Road Not Taken". It still hangs in my office, and every day reminds me of what is possible when you **TAKE ACTION.**

> *"Two roads diverged in a wood and I—I took the one less traveled by. And that has made all the difference."*

Chris Matthews of MSNBC's *Hardball* recently delivered a commencement address which provided specific advice to the graduates:

> "*. . . success cannot be assumed or taken for granted . . .*
> *everyone needs to leave the sidelines, get into the game and engage*
> *. . . in order to achieve one's hopes, dreams and goals.*"

There really is no other way. You are at that point now. In this book, I have pointed out which road for you to take. Now you need to leave the sidelines, and engage. **Take action now and make menopause the best years of your life!**

Selected Resources for
Additional Information

Informative and unbiased websites

- www.menopause.org
- www.webmd.com
- www.healthywomen.org
- www.redhotmamas.org
- www.asrm.org

Books

I have found these books on menopause to be useful and informative for my patients. Some of them may have, in part, areas of personal bias and controversy. In some areas, they may even disagree with some of my recommendations in this book. Pay attention to these differences. Also keep in mind the date of the publications and the rapidly changing "answers" to menopause issues.

Liu, J. H.; Gass, ML (eds). *Perimenopause: Practical Pathways in Obstetrics and Gynecology.* New York: McGraw-Hill. 2006.

Northrup, Christiane. *The Wisdom of Menopause.* New York: Bantam Books. 2001

Notelovitz, M; Tonnessen, D. *Menopause and Midlife Health.* New York: St. Martin's Press. 1993

Sheehy, Gail. *The Silent Passage: Menopause.* New York: Random House. 1992

Simpson, Kathryn; Bresden, Dale. *The Perimenopause and Menopause Workbook.* Oakland, California: New Harbinger Publications. 2006

Somers, Suzanne. *The Sexy Years.* New York: Crown Publishing. 2003

Vliet, Elizabeth L. *Screaming to Be Heard: Hormone Connections Women Suspect and Doctors Still Ignore.* New York: Evans and Company. 1995

Wingert, Pat; Kantrowitz, Barbara. *Is it Hot in Here? Or Is it Me? The Complete Guide to Menopause.* New York: Workman Publishing. 2006

Resources on Special Topics

Intimacy

Altman, Alan; Ashner, Laurie. *Making Love the Way We Used To . . . Or Better.* Chicago, Illinois: Contemporary Books. 2001

Cattral, Kim; Levinson, Mark. *Satisfaction: The Art of Female Orgasm.* New York: Warner Books. 2002

Crenshaw, TL. *The Alchemy of Love and Lust: How Our Sex Hormones Influence Our Relationships.* New York: Pocket Books. 1997

De Pavli, Carlo. *Secrets of Sexual Ecstasy: Pathways to Erotic Pleasure.* New York: Marlow & Company. 1996

Harley, Jr. William. *His Needs, Her Needs: Building An Affair Proof Marriage.* Grand Rapid, Michigan: Fleming H. Revell Books. 1986

Robbins, Anthony; Madanes, Cloé. *Ultimate Relationship Program.* www.ROBBINSMADANES.com 2005

Robbins, Anthony; Robbins, Sage. *Passion Project.* www.loversforlife-media.com. 2007

Schoen, Mark. *The Better Sex Video Series.* Chapel Hill, North Carolina: Sinclair Institute. 2005

Meditation/ Hypnosis

Kabat-Zinn, Jon. *Mindfulness Meditation: Cultivating the Wisdom of Your Body and Mind.* Niles, Illinois: www.nightingale.com

Kenyon, Tom. *The Ultimate Brain: Psychoacoustic Immersion.* Orcas, Washington: Acoustic Brain Research. www.tomkenyon.com 2006

Oakes, Luanne. *Sound Health, Sound Wealth.* Niles, Illinois: www.nightingale.com

———. *Spiritual Alchemy.* Niles, Illinois: www.nightingale.com

———. *Your Magical Divine Experiment.* Niles, Illinois: www.nightingale.com

Sulphen, Dick. *Hypnology: Transform Your Life With the Power of Self-Hypnosis.* Niles, Illinois: www.nightingale.com

Weil, A; Gurgevich, S. *Heal Yourself With Medical Hypnosis.* 2-CD set. www.DrWeil.com or 1–888–3DR-WEIL. 2006

Natural and Herbal Therapies

Blumenthal, Mark. *The ABC Clinical Guide to Herbs.* New York: Thieme. 2003

Duke, JA. *CRC Handbook of Medicinal Herbs.* Boca Raton, Florida. CRC Press, 1985

Low Dog, T, Mesozzi, MS. *Women's Health in Complementary and Integrative Medicine. A Clinical Guide.* St. Louis, Missouri: Elsevier. 2005

Tyler, VE. *The Honest Herbal.* Philadelphia: George F. Stickley Co. 1982

Weight Loss and Body Reconfiguration

Abdo, John; Dackman, Kenneth. *Body Engineering: How to Reconnect the Way you Look and Feel.* New York, New York: Berkley Publishing Group. 1997

Peeke, Pamela. *Body For Life for Women.* New York, New York: Rodale. 2005

Index

About the Authors

DR. HENRY HESS

Dr. Henry Hess received his Ph.D. in organic chemistry at Purdue University under one of the world's great chemists, 1979 Nobel Prize laureate Professor HC Brown. After completion of his doctorate, he became interested in natural medical therapies, leading to his study of medicine. He received his M.D. from New York Medical College, and trained as an obstetrician gynecologist at the University of Rochester School of Medicine. Dr. Hess currently serves as Associate Clinical Professor of Obstetrics and Gynecology at the University of Rochester School of Medicine.

Dr. Hess has practiced in all areas of OB/GYN for over 25 years with a special interest in menopause and perimenopause. He believes in the integrative approach—a blend of traditional and natural medicine, and this is the focus of *The Perfect Menopause: 7 Steps to the Best Time of Your Life*.

Dr. Hess is a board-certified obstetrician gynecologist, a certified menopause practitioner, and a certified hypnotherapist. He is known for his knowledge and expertise in natural therapies as well as hormonal therapies. Dr. Hess writes and lectures nationally on the topics of menopause, perimenopause, and other hormone problems.

TIFFANY FARRELL

Tiffany Farrell is a freelance medical writer specializing in women's health.

Order Form

Phone orders: (585) 234-0098

Online orders: http://www.theperfectmenopause.com
e-book: $10.95; trade paper book: $19.95.

Mail Orders: Westfall Park Publishing Group
2255 South Clinton Avenue
Rochester, New York 14618

Please send _____ copies of
The Perfect Menopause: 7 Steps to the Best Time of Your Life

$19.95 $_____

Shipping and Handling: United States standard: Add $2.50 for first book and $2.00
for each additional book (Allow 1-3 weeks for delivery)

Sales Tax: Add 4% for products shipped to New York addresses: $_____

Total: $_____

Payment:

❑ Check   ❑ Credit Card
❑ VISA   ❑ MasterCard

Credit Card #_____

Name on card: _____

Exp. date: _____

Signature: _____

Send to: (please print or type)

Name: _____

Address: _____

City: _____ State:_____ Zip: _____

E-mail:_____